M000248958

Keep Mothers and Babies Together
The Story of Dr. John Kennell

Karen Olness, MD, Carolyn Myers, PhD,
with Mary Hellerstein, MD

WITH THANKS TO

*Kalo Lockerby, Rachel Scheckter, Shanna Kralovic,
Susan McGrath, Susan Wood, Cristina Novoa,
Hakon Torjesen and the Kennell family for
their assistance in doing interviews, transcribing
interviews, providing interviews and editing.*

Praeclarus Press, LLC

www.PraeclarusPress.com

Praeclarus Press, LLC
2504 Sweetgum Lane
Amarillo, Texas 79124 USA
806-367-9950
www.PraeclarusPress.com

DISCLAIMER

The information contained in this publication is advisory only and is not intended to replace sound clinical judgment or individualized patient care. The author disclaims all warranties, whether expressed or implied, including any warranty as the quality, accuracy, safety, or suitability of this information for any particular purpose.

ISBN: 978-1-939807-31-1

Cover Design: Ken Tackett
Acquisition & Development: Kathleen Kendall-Tackett
Copy Editing: Chris Tackett
Layout & Design: Cornelia-Georgiana Murariu
Operations: Scott Sherwood

CONTENTS

Foreword

John Kennell's influence on my career was profound, and he probably had no idea that it occurred. Indeed, so much of John's influence on others is hidden under his characteristic modesty. In 1950, I was in the middle of my mixed-medicine internship at The University of Rochester and had decided to go into pediatrics, and wanted to be accepted at The Children's Hospital, Boston. I arranged for the interview and when I arrived, the chief, Dr. Charles Janeway, interviewed me. The first thing he said to me was that the recent chief resident there, John Kennell, was a graduate of the University of Rochester, and he was so good, that I must be good as well, and that he would accept me. John's long hand had boosted me to the place I wanted to be on the basis of his competence, not by any salesmanship on my part. Indeed, I never met John until some years later.

In 1955, as I was starting a program to educate pediatric residents and medical students about general pediatrics and child development at the Children's Hospital, Boston, I needed to learn what others were doing in this general field. The Family Heath Program, which John had initiated as part of the exciting curriculum reform at Case Western Reserve University, was by that time, world famous. I visited him. He was, as always, so accommodating and helpful. His knowledge of child development was far greater than I, or anyone on my staff had, but his building of the program around understanding of the family was exactly what I was looking for as the organizing principle of my program.

This was an era when several medical schools had developed "comprehensive care" programs to help medical students learn the need for understanding the social and mental health aspects of caring for patients. But none of the programs that I visited had such an explicit basis of the family as the most important factor for building a teaching and medical care program, as did

John's. I have not given him enough credit over the years for the inspiration that I took away from my visit to him as I tried to develop a program in which the family was the core social group for providing medical care, and in addition, the most important group influencing the development of children. John's low-key example of teaching child development in the context of families is a major contribution to the field of child development, and social medicine, one that John has never pushed aggressively. It is just not in John's character to be a self-promoter or salesman for his ideas. He lets time and the obvious success of his programs to do the promoting of his contributions.

Another experience that John had nothing to do with directly, but for which he was the inspiration behind, was demonstrated to me on a visit I made to Santiago, Chile for a continuing education course. Over the weekend, my host took me out to her father's large cattle ranch. I was surprised to see an area perhaps 50 feet by 50 feet with a tarp over it and hay on the ground. Under the tarp were three or four cows, one obviously in labor. I asked my host why. She said that a few years before they had cows deliver their calves alone in the barn, but had a lot of long labors and still births. On a visit by Marshall Klaus, he saw this and told them they needed to have the cows deliver with a few other cows outdoors in a comfortable setting. This was a translation of Klaus' and Kennell's work on the benefit of doulas in making human deliveries smoother. When they had done this, as I witnessed, the difficult labor and stillbirth rates dropped. I'm sure that John and Marshall never dreamed that their doula model would be so helpful to the cattle industry.

John's many contributions to human (and non-human) development, and its influence on many others, has been as hidden from him as was mine. It is time that he knows how much he has influenced so many, many others.

Robert J. Haggerty, MD
Professor of Pediatrics, University of Rochester
Past President, American Academy of Pediatrics
Past President, WT Grant Foundation

Preface

September 15, 2013 was a beautiful, sunny day in Cleveland, Ohio, as hundreds of people parked vehicles around the Case Western Reserve University campus and found their way to the Amasa Stone Chapel to attend the memorial service for John Hawkes Kennell. Soon, the large building was packed with doctors, nurses, former students, doulas, psychologists, parents, children, administrative assistants, research assistants, neighbors, patients now grown up, and, of course, his beloved wife Peggy, three children, five grandchildren, and nieces and nephews. All were John's friends, and most believed that he or she had a special relationship with Dr. Kennell. John was that kind of a man. He was a wonderful listener and would remember the ordinary details of the lives of the people he met.

The memorial service was long because so many people were eager to talk about this extraordinary man. Dr. Berry Brazelton wanted to speak; his physician would not allow him to travel, so he sent his colleague to speak for him. John's close colleagues in neonatology spoke. The Dean of the Medical School sent her husband to read her eulogy (She was at an NIH meeting). Representatives of DONA (Doulas of North America) gave beautiful talks about Kennell's contribution to DONA. One of John's sons, speaking on behalf of the Kennell family, gave a loving tribute to his father. The memorial service was truly a celebration of a long life, well lived (A few eulogies may be found in the chapter called Tributes). Following the service, the Kennell family hosted a gathering, during which the attendees shared memories and spent time looking at the photo display. There were lots of stories and lots of hugs. Young and old, men and women, adults and children, professional and nonprofessional—all were united by their positive memories of John Kennell. One former student wrote:

> Most did not know the extent of your fame, and you did
> not tell them. You remained true to yourself, embodying
> humility, generosity and, above all, love.

Introduction

Our first baby was born in December, 1965. How well I remember the onset of labor in the middle of the night, the ride to a university hospital at daylight with my husband driving. And as soon as we arrived, and were checked in, he was banished and I was alone. I had never met the nurses involved in my care; I did know the obstetrician, but she was present only at the actual delivery. And my husband sat in a stark waiting area for seven hours, also alone. I have only vague memories of the process I was guided through with one exception. The mandatory enemas seemed like torture for someone in active labor. I remember the joy in the middle of the afternoon when I heard the words, "It's a boy" and I heard him cry—a very special moment and my husband missed it.

My experience was typical for all mothers who had babies born in the hospital through most of the 20th century. Things began to change dramatically by the early 70s because of the work of two men—John Kennell and Marshall Klaus. They established the importance of early mother-infant attachment, and this led to rooming in for babies, and later, admission of family members to labor-and-delivery suites. This book is a story of John Kennell, a humble pediatrician, and how he came to focus his work on mothers and babies and support persons for women in labor, and also on grieving parents whose babies had died.

Today, Western families assume that family members can be present during labor and delivery, and cannot fathom how families were once excluded from this basic life experience. John Kennell was trained as a neonatologist. He became concerned about mothers who seemed disinterested in their newborn premature infants because they had almost no early contact with them. This led to his remarkable career.

In 1979, Dr. Kennell gave the George Armstrong Award lecture at the annual meeting of the Ambulatory Pediatric Association (Kennell, 1980). In this talk, he emphasized the need for scientists to choose the most promising components from our past and test these against our modern practices in long-term studies. He said, "Is it possible that we have discarded or overlooked treasures of evolutionary wisdom for human development in the rush of progress?" In his research, Dr. Kennell has been a leader in investigating old traditions in the care of infants, including breastfeeding, body contact between infant and mother, the presence of a supportive person during labor and delivery, and family participation in the care of sick children. His work has led to major changes in birthing practices in the United States, with increased early contact between mother and infant, and increased family involvement.

Were there antecedents of these outcomes in the early life of John Kennell? In preparing this biography we have reviewed scrapbooks and baby books, family letters, school reports, many photos, and more than 30 interviews with Dr. Kennell and others close to him. We have organized the chapters of this book according to the sequence of his life with the exception of several statements written by colleagues who have known him well. Wherever possible, we have quoted his own words in describing the events of his life.

SECTION I

EDUCATION AND WORK
IN CLEVELAND

Chapter 1
THE EARLY YEARS

John Kennell was born on January 9, 1922, in Reading, Pennsylvania. This first-born child entered a large extended family and was welcomed with great attention and recognition. His detailed baby book, kept meticulously by his mother, Doris Hawks Kennell, notes that the family received 16 plants and flowers; 3 gifts of fruit, nuts, and candy; 92 baby gifts, including three that were money; and 63 letters and telegrams in honor of his birth. A letter from his uncle, Will Hawks, written on January 13, 1922, said:

> Dear Doris,
>
> That was very pleasing news contained in a card received yesterday. "John Hawks Kennell." I like that name. If the young man proves as good in every way as the man after whom he is named, he will have no difficulty in passing successfully through the world. I not only want to congratulate yourself and husband on the addition to your family, but thank you for giving him the name of "John." It will prove a winner. It is nearly a hundred years (March 31, 1825) since his great grandfather appeared on the scene. It is probable that within a few months his first baby picture will be taken. Don't forget to remember Uncle Will and Aunt Helen. The grandparents in Rochester were very "mum," not even a hint being given

in any letter from them as to "expectations." I hope that both the father and mother are "doing well" and are contented in Reading. Neither Aunt Helen nor myself have enjoyed good health this winter. Planned to go to New York, but are not sure now whether we will go or not. Bess was up here for Thanksgiving. She is well and happy. Have had severe weather the past week but it is clear and cold today with lots of snow. Hoping that the Kennell family including Young John will prosper, and with love to you all from both of us. From your Aff.

Uncle Will

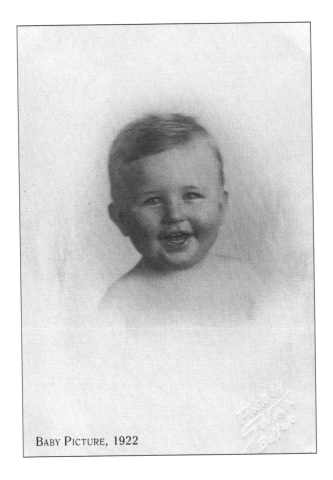

BABY PICTURE, 1922

A letter from his maternal grandmother, Ida Parker Hawkes, written on January 11, 1922, said:

> Dearest Dorrie,
>
> I can assure you we were pleased to get the telegram at ten o'clock this morning telling us of the good news. How I wish I could come in to see you today, and the little man.
>
> I am just as anxious now to get Carlyle's letter as I was to get the telegram.
>
> . . . Grandmother Kennell just called us a few minutes ago and she is as glad as we are. She said she would try to get over before many days. Were you disappointed that the baby was a boy? Your doctor was wrong all around, wasn't he? . . . Now you write me what day I better come. I don't want to come very long before you come home for I would rather have the time after you are home than while you are in the hospital. If you get along as we all hope you will, you will be able to write after a few days, but don't try to be smart. Just keep quiet as long as you can. And don't have much company. I do hope you can nurse the little fellow. How I want to see you both today. Now be a good girl and don't hesitate to ask your nurse to do anything you want done.
>
> > Lots of love to you.
> > Pa and Mama

. . .

John Kennell lived in a poorer section of Buffalo, New York, until he was of school age. The family, including one sister, lived in the lower flat of a two-story house. He recalls that the childless couple living in the upstairs flat was very friendly to him. He also remembered seeing many rats around the garbage cans containing hops (this was the time of Prohibition) outside and also in their basement. The rats didn't seem to faze John Kennell, but he described two childhood experiences which did:

> I remember I had a tricycle and I was so happy with it. We lived on a long street which intersected with a busier street. I was told to go to the end of it with my tricycle and turn around. One day, there was a big truck stopped in our street. It might have been a delivery truck or a furniture truck. The two drivers were sitting in the truck and I was just staring at them. I think my staring bothered them, and the sons of guns came and told me to go. I didn't leave, and then they tied my wheel to the frame of the truck. I remember them being unfriendly toward me. Nothing further happened, but I guess it scared me. Another event that scared me, when I was three or four years old, happened in a nearby store where we would go to get small things like bread. I don't know why, perhaps I was tired, but one day I sort of leaned against the glass front and it fell or broke. I felt very guilty about that.

Before marriage, John's resourceful paternal grandmother had worked as a traveling seamstress--an unfamiliar profession today. She would stay in a home for several days, making clothing, and thereby earn her keep. Her parents had come from England. John's paternal grandfather had a farm near Rochester, New York. He came from several generations of farmers in the area. There was a large house, but no indoor plumbing, and water came from a well. His father, Carlyle Kennell, was born on the farm. John's grandfather died before John was born, so his father worked to put himself through high school and college. His grandmother continued to live on the farm until she died in 1933, and John Kennell spent a great deal of time there, especially during summers. He describes his paternal grandmother as "unbelievably devoted to me." She probably had only three or four years of schooling, but somehow learned to read and write. She would read to John every night. As far as he was concerned as a

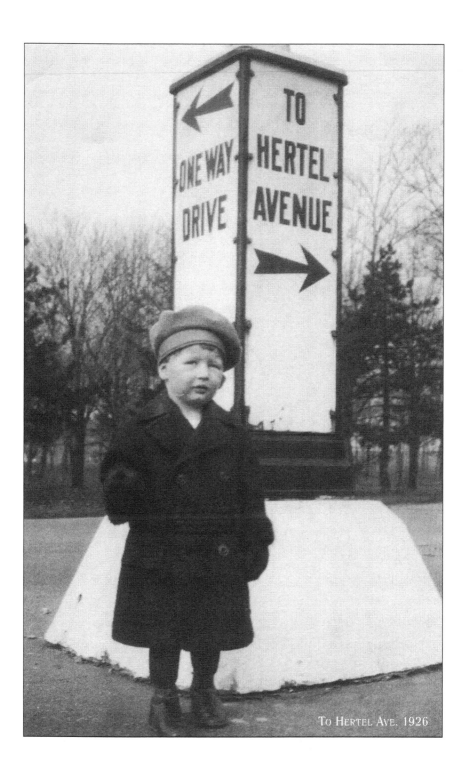

To Hertel Ave. 1926

little boy, she knew everything there was to know about the world. In her house, she had a piano and two organs, which were of great interest to him. She was known as someone who was good at attending childbirths, and sometimes, she would tell John about the births the next morning.

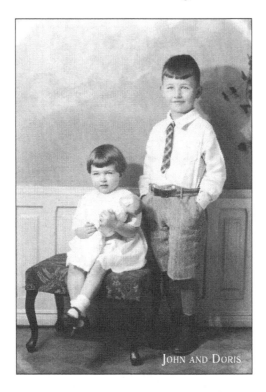

JOHN AND DORIS

John was a thin child and his grandmother tried to fatten him. She fed him well, including giving him extra honey. The Kennell grandparents raised gladiola and honey bees on their 13-acre farm, and John could not understand how they could survive just through sales of gladiolas and honey. Yet his father managed to attend the University of Rochester, as did his mother: the first members of their families to be university graduates. His mother was an English teacher for a few years before she married. Throughout childhood, he and his sister were expected to do well in school. John felt that this instilled in him the desire and concept to progress intellectually and to get to a place where he could apply that intellectual background.

During his visits to the farm, John Kennell also spent time with his paternal uncle and aunt, Everett and Harriet Kennell, who lived across the street from the farm. His uncle was a high school teacher who worked on the farm in the summers. John remembers being involved in plowing, haying, and picking fruit. One could get a few pennies for picking boxes of raspberries and currents. He recalls that his uncle made him a hand plow out of a toy baby carriage. He added automobile engine parts to the hand plow, and John made noises to pretend that it actually had a gas engine. It was so convincing that one of his young friends believed it was a real engine.

His uncle also gave him a crystal set. Kennell remembers hearing a broadcast celebrating Charles Lindberg's flight across the Atlantic at a time when none of the Kennell neighbors had a radio. At least once a week during the summers, his grandmother would organize a picnic that he enjoyed along with his grandparents and uncle. His father, mother, and sister would come to the farm from Buffalo on some weekends to visit John and to garden. He recalls "working" in the fields with his little rake as he moved alongside his father and uncle, and he remembers washing up with them after the work was done. John believes that his interest in gardening, plants, and nature evolved from the many discussions with this uncle and his father at the farm.

Because John's grandmother was often busy with work on the farm, John notes that he was free to explore on his own quite often. He describes how he enjoyed climbing pine trees and hanging upside down, exploring a quarry and a creek, and catching turtles in the creek. His uncle raised collie dogs. One of John's favorite collies was named Barkus. When Barkus fell through the ice in a quarry one winter, and could not be rescued, John cried for two or three days.

John's beloved grandmother died when he was 10 years old. After her death, he no longer spent time on the farm. His father and uncle rented out the house and careless tenants started a fire that destroyed the house. John continued his close relationship with his paternal uncle, who was always very interested in John's medical school work, and who would ask him many questions.

> My mother's family, the Parker family, was a very bright, active, stimulating group of people who lived in Georgetown, New York, a tiny community. There were four Parker sisters, with John's grandmother Ida being the oldest. They lived on a farm on a hill above Main Street, and as they walked to school they happened to pass the home of Ida's future husband, Charles Hawks. In the age of prohibition "my mother was embarrassed to report that they raised hops to be sold for making beer."

Charles Hawks had a plant nursery in Rochester, New York, the area where John's mother (the second of three children), grew up. Susan B. Anthony was a big influence in the area and John feels this may have helped prompt his mother to attend college. To him, she appeared both beautiful and a pioneer. Charles moved with Ida to Milwaukee in the early 1930s. Going to Milwaukee was a long trip from Buffalo. For this reason, young John Kennell did not spend as much time with these grandparents as he did with his paternal grandmother.

John recalls his father "was a very conscientious and devoted father, always attentive." His father could speak well, but was a particularly good listener, a trait mentioned frequently about John. His father was a traveling insurance salesman, who was transferred from Reading, Pennsylvania, to Buffalo, New York, shortly before John's birth. He had two weeks of vacation a year.

After the Kennells were able to purchase a car, most of their travel and vacations were between Buffalo and Rochester. When John was about 8 years old, the family began a series of summer vacations at a little lake in central New York State. His mother's older sister, Laura Barss, and her son, Ted, and the Kennell family would rent a cottage there for two weeks. Laura's husband,

Howard, and John's father would visit for a few days. Ted Barss was John's age and the two boys were good friends. The Kennells continue a connection with his cousin to the present.

The Kennell family had many family gatherings with the extended Parker family. The Parker family traced back to a Mr. Parker, who came across the Atlantic on the Mayflower. One of the family members, Philo Parker (first cousin of Kennell's mother), had spent a long time in China. He developed business for Standard Oil Company of New York in China and Hong Kong. Among other positions, he later became the chairman of the Standard Vacuum Oil Company.

During vacations, the Kennell family sometimes visited the Barss family in Oregon. Howard P. Barss was a pioneer in botany and plant pathology, and a great inspiration to John's son, Jack.

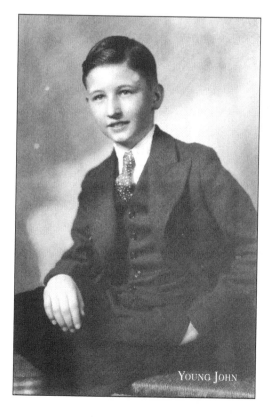

YOUNG JOHN

For almost 40 years, Howard was head of a department of the same name at Oregon State University in Corvallis. He served in many positions, including Chairman of the Division of Biological Sciences of the USDA Graduate School during WWII. While John himself spent very little time with Howard Barss, he always found it "exciting and educational."

When John was of school age, the family moved to a rental house. During the Depression, there was no further home building and everyone was poor. The house was in a development where there were many children and they had access to a large field. In the spring and winter, this area was full of ponds that froze. John's parents strung up lights so that skating could take place at night. John learned to play hockey. He also played pick-up football and baseball with neighborhood boys, and ran errands for neighbors. He played with his sister, Doris, who was two years younger. When she developed scarlet fever, the family home was quarantined for 2 months because she failed to develop the characteristic skin peeling. During this period, John was also confined to the family home area. It was winter and there was much snow, as is usual in Buffalo. During the quarantine period, John became an expert at building igloos by himself in the backyard.

The Kennell family had a fox terrier, and John enjoyed playing outside with him. When the fox terrier died, he obtained a cat which learned to ride on his shoulder as he rode his bicycle. Kennell recalls turning over rocks in the fields near their home so the cat could catch mice.

John Kennell said that as they got older, he and his friends spent much time at the railroad tracks and on a nearby train bridge. For several years, there was a "hobo" camp near these railroad tracks and the hobos built fires most evenings.

Across the swampy fields behind the Kennell house, there was a busy highway and a cross street with less traffic and a stop sign. Drivers were not accustomed to stop signs; it was not unusual to have their baseball or football games interrupted by tragic car accidents caused by drivers who whizzed

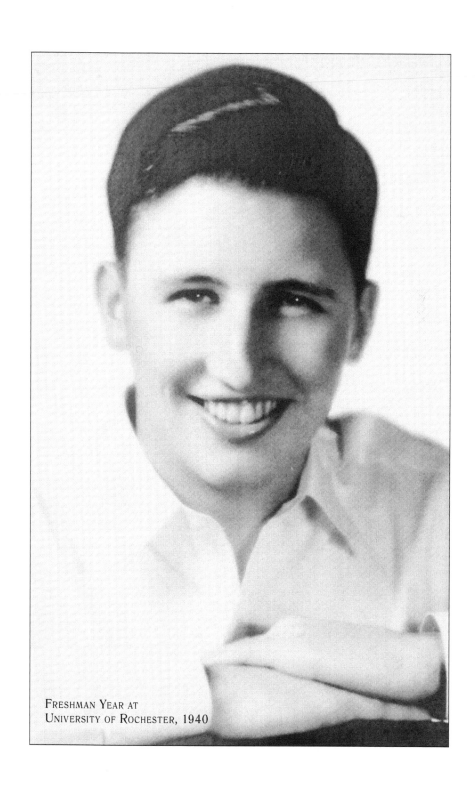

FRESHMAN YEAR AT
UNIVERSITY OF ROCHESTER, 1940

through the stop sign. One day, a visiting cousin, who was four years older, took John and his sister to this crossing to write down the license numbers of cars that went through the stop signs. They recorded several pages of license numbers over three or four hours. They mailed the list of numbers to the police department, but never received a response.

John felt he was fortunate to attend a relatively new high school with mostly young, enthusiastic teachers. At a 50th reunion, two of his teachers were able to come. They claimed that John's classmates were all good children and that they didn't have much trouble with them. Truly, the worst thing the whole class could think of was that one classmate, Willis Whiting, was once caught smoking in the seventh grade—but he turned out "good."

Reflecting upon his choice of pediatrics, John cites experiences from his own childhood. While few people had jobs during the Depression, his father continued to work, though his salary was reduced over and over again. Consequently, they were able to have a pediatrician. John remembers that pediatricians seemed less busy then. When he was sick at home, his doctor would stop and take time to play a game or work on a puzzle with him. That made a great impression!

On account of being a Boy Scout for a long time, John's first summer job was serving as a counselor at Y camps; a rewarding experience in working with children. Even in his first year of college, it became clear to John that he would like to go to medical school. Then, as detailed in the next chapter, John's pre-med and medical school during WWII, was paid for by the military. Payback included working away from the ivory tower. He was sent to a very, very busy clinic in Norfolk, Virginia, and had very heavy responsibilities for the care of an enormous number of children. It exposed him to so many of their real-life dilemmas.

Note: See Appendices: Essay on Selling Magazines and Valedictory Speech.

Chapter 2
HIGHER EDUCATION

John Kennell thrived at the University of Rochester and felt fortunate to join Phi Beta Kappa. He learned how to bypass the many wild fraternity parties by finding secluded places in the stacks of the Rochester library where he could diligently study. John did not experience WWII first hand because he was attending college and medical school. However, he enrolled in the military and was grateful that they paid the tuition for medical school.

Most medical schools were shortening the training period by eliminating vacation time and lengthening training days. John Kennell was in one of these accelerated programs and recalls having one five-to-seven day break between the first and second years, and again between the second and third years of training. Many of the experienced clinical faculty had been drafted, so there were fewer faculty available to teach medical students. John Kennell had great respect and admiration for George Whipple, Dean of the Rochester School of Medicine. He was a Nobel Prize winning pathologist who made important discoveries related to anemia. Dean Whipple spoke to medical students often and insisted that they spend an hour each day in the gym for recreation. He also told students not to read the newspaper or listen to the radio. John remarks that they didn't follow these last two things too well.

John recalls that anatomy was heavily emphasized during the first year of medical school and that there seemed to be undue emphasis on dissecting the hands and fingers compared to dissection of the thorax. He felt that he had not had the opportunity to adequately understand the anatomy of the heart and great vessels. He regretted this later during his pediatric residency when there was a new interest in, and emphasis on, congenital cardiac disease in infants.

Physiology was a very appealing area of study for John. During World War II, there was great concern about the effects of altitude sickness on soldiers, and medical schools were asked to research this problem. Medical students at the University of Rochester were allowed to participate in research involving a pressure chamber (to simulate altitude changes) and measurements of physiologic changes. This was one of John's first research experiences, and he found it both interesting and inspiring. One professor, Dr. Adolf, taught about fluids and electrolytes. He expected his students to do their homework, and he spent a lot of time getting them to figure out answers that were not always correct. He was probably the students' least favorite teacher due to his teaching style. However, later, most students came to believe he was the best teacher because he had really made them think.

The Head of Pediatrics at the University of Rochester Medical School was an older pediatrician whose clinical activities were limited. His many lectures on the composition of infant formulas did not inspire the students of Kennell's generation. Another pediatrician in private practice, Dr. William Bradford, spent half days in the hospital and did a lot of teaching. He also did research on pertussis. When he became aware that John was interested in pediatrics, he helped him select an internship. He remained available and encouraging when John returned for visits to Rochester.

One classmate, Kenneth Holt, was brought to the U.S. from England by the Rockefeller Foundation, which was supporting a small number of promising British medical students away from the dangerous situation in London. Holt and Kennell were good friends, and he later facilitated John's sabbatical in England. John remained in contact with many of his classmates over the years and attended reunions regularly. John Kennell attended medical school during tumultuous times and was well aware of the stresses for colleagues and friends who had family members in the military overseas. Working on an emergency ambulance throughout his fourth year of medical school, he recalled that many women attempted suicide upon hearing the news that their husbands were returning after years of overseas duty. He noted that none of these women died.

Fifty students were in his graduating class of 1946. Several had dropped out, or been delayed by contracting tuberculosis or rheumatic fever. All who had been in the U.S. Army ASTP and Navy V-12 during part of medical school were required to take rotating internships. Following graduation, John Kennell went to the Children's Hospital in Boston for his pediatrics internship.

Prior to the conclusion of medical school, in early 1946, John Kennell was invited by a professor of radiology at his medical school to volunteer to participate as an observer and helper in the pending Bikini atom bomb tests. He began his pediatric internship in April, but was released a month later for six weeks to join the group from the University of Rochester who participated in the Bikini atom bomb tests. For young Dr. Kennell, this was an amazing experience. First, he traveled more than he had ever traveled, flying to the west coast, and then traveling by hospital ship to the Bikini area. The U.S. government had arranged for thousands of observers, including some Russian scientists. John Kennell met many outstanding scientists, and there were lectures every day on some aspect of the planned atomic testing. He and other medical students worked every day in moving supplies to several captured battleships. During the actual atomic testing, Kennell was 26 miles from the testing area. The tests were successfully accomplished in June 1946, and Kennell then returned to his duties at Boston Children's Hospital.

Living in Boston was a great change from living in western New York. John didn't know anyone when he arrived in Boston, and he was much younger than many of the other trainees who had spent years in military service. His pay was room and board, and $27 dollars every three months. He shared a room with another intern. Hours were long, and the work was hard, but

John sensed that he was there during a "glorious period" in medicine. For example, antibiotics were in early use, having been made generally available at the conclusion of the war.

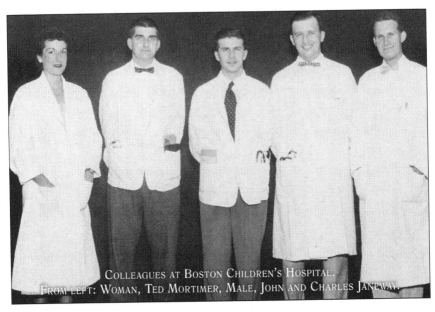

COLLEAGUES AT BOSTON CHILDREN'S HOSPITAL.
FROM LEFT: WOMAN, TED MORTIMER, MALE, JOHN AND CHARLES JANEWAY.

In pediatrics there were many new discoveries related to diagnosis and treatment. Cardiac surgery was just beginning at Boston Children's Hospital, and John Kennell, the intern, felt that he was working among giants. He rubbed shoulders with many young physicians who later became famous. These included Fred Robbins (who later encouraged him to go to Cleveland), Jack Metcoff, William Wallace (who had been in the army for a long time in North Africa), Charles A. Janeway, Ralph Wedgewood, and Sydney Gellis. There were also weekly conferences at Brigham and Women's Hospital, where many speakers enlightened John and the rest of the medical community.

During this time John Kennell was storing away observations about hospital traditions that later came to bother him a great deal.

At the Children's Hospital in Boston, like most or all the big hospitals for children in the U.S. in 1946, parents were not allowed in the hospital except to visit on Saturday afternoon. I was warned by everybody that this was what wise senior physicians had decided. Because it was so upsetting to children to see their parents, they thought it was best not to have them come but two hours on one day each week.

Parents were allowed in only when the child was admitted, on Saturdays and when the child was discharged, or if the child died. At that time, death was a common occurrence on the divisions where I worked; there was a big diarrhea epidemic that was highly fatal. What the senior physicians had suggested was true. When the parents came, some children would have diarrhea and some would vomit. It was not uncommon for the children to develop a fever. The parents hardly knew their little children and the little children hardly knew their parents.

When the children were a bit older, they showed a lot of anger, but also a lot of love and enthusiasm, along with a great deal of crying and stress when the parents had to leave. In many ways it was a cruel prison-like situation.

At this time, before continuous IV fluids were used in pediatrics, an interminable number of feverish babies and children required IV treatments throughout the day, totally exhausting all those involved. Protocols were also scarce. Added to the intense experience of children with diarrhea came the necessity, and for John, the great learning opportunity to talk with the parents of the many babies who died. He encouraged them to call him if they wanted. They did. He listened.

John's interest in appreciating the world from the child's point of view was furthered upon meeting a professor, Dr. Romano. Medical school had incorporated almost no psychiatry. Now he occasionally joined a classmate at Peter Bent Brigham for breakfast. Dr. Romano also would be there, and would be recruited afterward to start the psychiatry department at Rochester.

Internship days were also personally rewarding for John. There he met Margaret Lloyd, his "Peggy," who would be his greatest support for the rest of his life. She had lost both parents at an early age and was passed among relatives. The Johnstown flood of 1936 provided a terrifying experience,

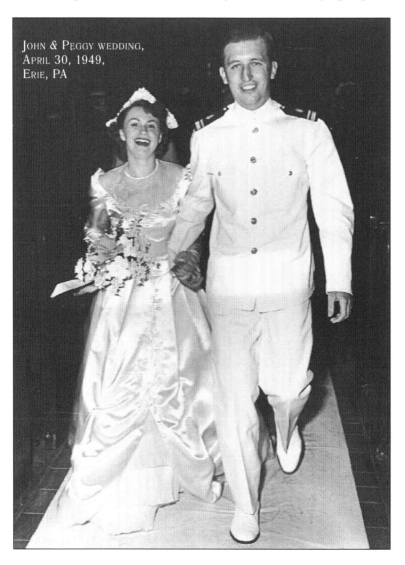

JOHN & PEGGY WEDDING,
APRIL 30, 1949,
ERIE, PA

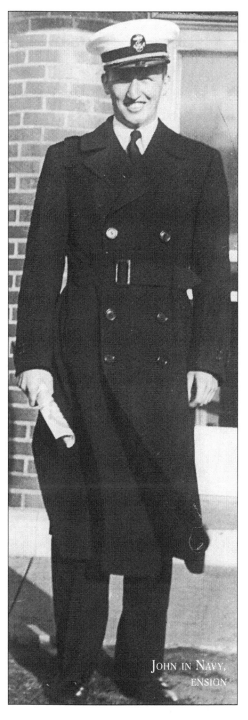

JOHN IN NAVY,
ENSIGN

during which she was separated from her grandparents. However, she also learned people could be kind and helpful.

There were happier times while she lived with an uncle in her teen years. An aunt from Erie, Pennsylvania, encouraged this lively young lady to take up nursing. Throughout, Peggy came to have great compassion for the sufferings of children, and graduated into the nursing staff in surgery. Thriving in the operating room, she became assistant head nurse—and one of John's pals.

John began his pay-back responsibilities to the military by working at the children's hospital in Chelsea Naval Hospital in Massachusetts, and then spent a couple months doing the difficult task of returning long-dead soldiers, sailors, and Marines to their families. It was upsetting and disruptive for virtually everyone involved. Once again he was exposed to enormous grief and women who attempted suicide.

In the end, the military transferred him to be in charge of a busy children's clinic at the Naval Station in Norfolk, Virginia. There was one toughened navy nurse who John said, "blamed most things on the weather and that seemed to comfort a lot of people." He slept in the barracks where pilots slept, so he knew about the losses and burns due to the emergence of the jet engine. The jet engines were so powerful relative to gas engines that they would "pull right off the airplane and the plane would crash" during landing.

The Norfolk experience was an auspicious time for John. He had been corresponding with Peggy, and occasionally seeing her in Washington D.C. or New York City. They were then engaged and married in the fall of 1948, in Erie, Pennsylvania. They returned to Norfolk for a short time. John felt so happy that the woman he married had "such a wonderful friendliness." Her great attentiveness and relationship to children helped him realize important aspects about his own profession. Throughout his life, John was lavish in his admiration for all the home and civic responsibilities that Peggy undertook, always with an outgoing, generous spirit. It was undoubtedly John's own generous spirit that Dr. Janeway noticed.

While in Norfolk, John was invited by Dr. Janeway to become an assistant resident at Boston Children's Hospital. He accepted. This required turning down a pediatric cardiology residency at Hopkins, a difficult decision.

During his very busy residency, John became Chief Resident of the Outpatient Department, Chief Resident of the Medical Service, and spent some months in a junior faculty position. He came to be known for his skills as a problem solver. John Kennell experienced many influences during residency. One was Charles Janeway, who was doing research on nephrotic syndrome. It impressed John how kind and thoughtful he was with every child and parent. Even when incredibly busy, he would spend precious time with a parent in need. In addition, Dr. Janeway, with his great foresight, recruited Roswell Gallagher to set up a program in adolescent medicine, before that was common. Similarly, he recruited Julius Richmond to be head of psychiatry at Children's. Finally, at this time Harold Stuart at the nearby Harvard School of Public Health was developing the growth charts that have been a boon for the practice of pediatrics.

During John's final year of chief residency, a visiting psychiatrist, Dane Prugh, began testing the effects of involving Child Life people on one of the divisions. He also was presenting the concept of bringing parents into the hospital. This was a radical idea because parents were considered harmful. During John's medical school, even medical students and interns were not allowed to enter the premature unit. As described in the next chapter, all these ideas were about to be challenged.

Note: Quotations in this chapter came from interviews of John Kennell, conducted by Dr. Mary Hellerstein.

Chapter 3
EARLY RESPONSIBILITIES AND
OBSERVATIONS IN CLEVELAND

Impressive changes were underway in 1952, when Dr. Kennell arrived in Cleveland. A new suite for premature infants opened. A radical new Medical School Curriculum, envisioned by Dean Wearn, was being created. It included a new Family Clinic that would involve Dr. Kennell. The pediatric faculty was small and mostly new. Dr. Kennell began his work as director of the new premature nursery. It had large windows that allowed observation of the nursery. Most neonatal units in the United States did not have such windows at that time. He was also responsible for newborn babies at MacDonald House, and for babies under 2 years of age. To say he was very busy while learning his way around a new hospital system is an understatement. Other responsibilities included participation in meetings pertaining to the new curriculum, and being an assistant to Dr. Sam Spector, the interim chairman of the Department of Pediatrics. Dr. Kennell noted that "Dr. Spector was a remarkable clinician and an excellent teacher. He just got better as the years went on. Students and residents loved to see him, and he always had good ideas for them." He became the Head of Pediatrics at the University of Chicago, and always remained a friend to Dr. Kennell.

Dr. William Wallace was soon recruited to lead the Department of Pediatrics and to become part of the curriculum revision. He had participated in building a flame photometer back at Boston Children's Hospital and proceeded to build one in Cleveland. It was invaluable for measuring serum sodium in the parade of children with diarrhea and dehydration. Today, such instruments are so common that it's hard to appreciate their great impact. Dr. Wallace was a scientist who went on to promote and strengthen academic investigations within the department.

One tradition in those early days that greatly appealed to Dr. Kennell was the doctor's dining room. Doctors would stand outside the entrance and would be seated according to how they had lined up. He felt "it mixed people up wonderfully," and was an excellent way for scientists and clinicians to casually meet and discuss students, committees, and future plans for both pediatrics and the medical school.

Premature Babies, Their Mothers, and Families

At that time, at least in the developed world, the absolute rule was that parents were not allowed into the premature nursery because so many deaths were due to infection. Before antibiotics, these infections were catastrophic, but there were also many deaths from infections after the advent of antibiotics. Although, Dr. Kennell and the senior neonatal nurses initiated a gradual process to encourage mothers to look at their infants through the observation windows, this was in conflict with guidelines in the leading book on neonatology by Clement Smith in Boston. Whenever he would come to town to visit his sister in Chagrin Falls, the head nurse, Jane Cable, ruled out visitors for three days.

Dr. Kennell, nurses, and residents often heard comments from the mothers who were observing their babies. Their comments and appearances reflected their sadness and despair because they could not touch or hold their premature babies. Dr. Kennell said:

That was what led us to gradually let parents into the nursery
. . . When we did so, we kept track of things closely and

we were very fussy with mothers about how much they scrubbed. Because of their elation at getting close to their babies, they scrubbed very diligently and followed our rules very carefully. At first they could just stand by the isolette and observe their infants. Then we had them scrub more and they could touch their babies. Depending on a baby's condition and a mother's cooperation, we were able to allow the mother to increase her time and activities with her baby. We never had an infection.

Dr. Kennell and his staff found that mothers of the premature babies related to their infants differently than did mothers of full-term babies. All the mothers of preemies were anxious about touching their infants and would just touch with their fingertips at first, whereas a mother with a full-term baby would quickly use one or both hands and hold the baby firmly. Dr. Kennell elaborated:

We observed the mothers at various times and noted that they would use only one finger the first time, and then more than one after two or three visits. In the beginning, they used only their fingertips . . . We considered this very unusual behavior . . . Still it's understandable that the tiny baby's environment made the mother nervous and cautious . . . Usually there was IV fluid running into the baby, and oxygen being given, and other interventions. If the mother kept visiting as the baby got larger, she became more confident and would put her hand into the isolette and stroke the baby's body, especially if we said it was okay or encouraged them.

Dr. Kennell said he was initially cautious about allowing mothers to spend time with their premature infants. He would check on their hand washing and behavior. Gradually, the nursery became more open to parents, but it was inconvenient for some maternity nurses to bring mothers over to the premature nursery. Dr. Kennell observed that the "staff" mothers were not brought to the premature nursery as often as the private-paying mothers. "Staff" patient was a term used throughout University Hospitals at that time for patients from indigent families, who did not have a private physician. He explained,

> There was a continuous struggle to get every mother over to the nursery as soon as we could. However, the mothers who did not have private doctors also came to see their babies and became very devoted to them. I don't think we found any overall bonding differences between those two groups.

Dr. Kennell added, "The wonderful head nurse in that premature nursery, Jane Cable, and I and the other nurses became proud of how well mothers did with their babies."

Although Dr. Kennell and the nursing staff saw the advantages of early visitation with premature infants, they never wrote a paper about it. He said,

> We worked out a pattern for mothers based on keeping track of what a whole series of mothers did. For most of our studies we used an old movie camera. We took photos and analyzed them, and from that we would get data about what mothers did. The literature was so heavy on not ever letting parents into the nursery because of infection that we were cautious not to publicize this.

Dr. Kennell also became increasingly concerned about the lack of support for the largely African American families of the premature babies and other newborns. He began meeting with mothers of the so-called staff patients in groups, two or three times a week in 1952, and quickly realized that there were two types of mothers. One group consisted of grandmothers and their daughters, who originally came from the south during World War II for work. The young mothers had close ties with their mothers, who provided them guidance, and also provided support and guidance to the group. The advice was usually sound, although, often different from what pediatricians were recommending. Other new mothers in the group lacked the close family ties, and often did not have a husband or mother for support. Many of these needed a lot of information.

Dr. Kennell observed that, "Those sessions were particularly helpful if there was an experienced grandmother or mother who could inform the others. I thought that was very valuable for the women, and I learned a lot that I wouldn't have known otherwise."

Breastfeeding

On the home front, Dr. Kennell's own wife was breastfeeding their first child. He confessed, regarding his experience with his own baby, that "a lot of things came up that were educational for [him] later on."

At first, Dr. Kennell noted that all the African American mothers on the staff service were breastfeeding. Unfortunately, when prepared formula came along, in spite of the limited income of these families, they almost all switched to formula. He stated, "I guess in 2007 there are a great many descendants of those families who are still giving formula in spite of all the arguments in favor of breastfeeding." He explained further:

> In the early years, we had some excellent nurses working in these nurseries who were not RNs, but they were very, very good. They really could relate to all mothers, but particularly to the African Americans. Then University Hospitals had a change in the leadership of nursing. I believe it was a male nurse who decided that all the nurses in the nursery had to be highly trained. So there were a great many new graduates from the Francis Paine Bolton School of Nursing who came in and replaced these women who were so knowledgeable, and so helpful to doctors, as well as to the parents. The

replacement nurses didn't know half of what they should have understood, particularly about breastfeeding. Their plan was to offer a bottle with formula every three-to-four hours. Ironically, by the end of that first summer, I think all the new nurse graduates had resigned and taken other positions. The nursery was left with recruits who did not have as much experience and tolerance as the ones who had been dismissed earlier.

Unfortunately, nurses who worked on these units, and who were trained in the practice of bottle-feeding, frequently decided not to breastfeed when they themselves had babies. Dr. Kennell stated:

> The low time for breastfeeding at Babies and Children's hospital, in Cleveland and in the United States, was 1960. While the breastfeeding rate has improved, it is not yet sufficient.

Resuscitation of Newborns

Another responsibility for Dr. Kennell took place in the 8th-floor delivery suite at MacDonald Hospital (the maternity hospital). That hospital was staffed with obstetricians, but when a baby needed resuscitation, a pediatrician would be called. Not only was the physical process of getting to the suite an arduous trek down seven floors of Babies and Children's, and up eight floors at MacDonald, but there was also no plan or place for the resuscitation—except a broom closet. All these obstacles would ultimately be remedied, but the intense episodes among the mops always remained fresh in Dr. Kennell's mind. In time, the obstetricians came to invite Dr. Kennell to some of their meetings, and to present cases. For a great many years it seemed he was requested to look after a few babies, particularly from the west side of Cleveland.

Tonsillectomies and Parent Access

Dr. Kennell was also alert to the needs of older children:

> In the 1950s I was aware that children were being admitted
> in increasing numbers to a division that was set aside for
> children having a tonsillectomy and adenoidectomy. These
> children would be in cribs designed for children up to 6 to
> 10 years of age. There was no staying overnight . . . This
> division for tonsillectomy and adenoidectomy was a new
> development . . . Previously, in Cleveland, pediatricians had
> done many tonsillectomies in the home. There were deaths
> . . . so there was more and more emphasis on doing these
> procedures in the hospital with anesthesiologists . . .
>
> As the number of tonsillectomies increased in the hospital,
> there were more and more requests by mothers to stay with
> their children. They were turned down repeatedly. For a
> period of time, several of us would suggest to the mother that
> she could bring in a sleeping bag and sleep under the crib
> (this was after checking with the nurses). Mothers readily
> available were really roughing it because it was a hard floor
> and there were no toileting facilities. But bless them; more
> and more mothers began to request this option. I mention
> this because the parental requests eventually led to changes
> in hospital policy. I saw a clear advantage for the child if the
> mother could somehow stay with him or her.

Dr. Kennell describes one particular case:

> Sometime in the 50s or 60s I had a family with several
> children who were my patients. As I got to know the mother
> better, I learned that she had lived in Babies and Children's
> Hospital for a long period, 6 to 8 months as a child. Her

mother or her grandmother had been with her almost every day. Well, I didn't appreciate that part when she first told me. I couldn't imagine that there wouldn't be affects on a child of 3 staying in the hospital that long. So it was astounding to find out that she had become a very good mother, and I wondered how that happened. Now the importance of her mother and grandmother being with her became clear. It was allowed because her uncle was a physician who referred patients to Babies and Children's Hospital, and that gave him more influence. He insisted that her mother and grandmother remain with her, and so this excellent young mother displayed no evidence of long-term trauma.

Note: John Kennell quotations were taken from unpublished interviews conducted by Mary Hellerstein, MD on February 16, 2007, March 21, 2007, June 13, 2007, July 18, 2007, and August 23, 2007, and an interview by Dr. Carl Doershuk on October 30, 2006.

Chapter 4

TEACHING IN THE FAMILY CLINIC AND CLINICAL SCIENCES

Included in the new medical school curriculum was a program to teach medical students about families. Each student was assigned to a pregnant woman who was being followed on the staff service at MacDonald Hospital (the maternity hospital). The student was to follow the mother and her baby for four years. The objectives of this program were: 1) to give students a sense of the professional responsibilities of a physician; 2) to allow students contact with patients early in their training and thereby gain an understanding of the complexities of the patient-physician relationship; and 3) to help them learn about child development and family dynamics. As with most new programs, difficulties are frequently encountered. But this program ultimately survived and thrived for 50 years.

Students assigned to visit mothers during their prenatal visits would find these visits challenging. Dr. Kennell wrote:

> The students didn't know what to say to the mothers, and the mothers didn't know what to say to the students. Very often the student and mother would sit in the clinic sometimes far apart … usually with little communication. You had all sorts of different personality combinations, and you can imagine

how difficult it was if a very assertive mother was paired with a beginning student.

Next, students would be notified when mothers were admitted to the hospital in labor, and told to observe the labor-and-delivery process, including the mother's first contact with her baby. Dr. Kennell commented that for most students, this was the first delivery they had ever witnessed, and it was exciting for them. Students also were fascinated by everything that happened in the hospital, with the result that the Family Clinic program became a very valuable introduction to many aspects of medicine.

After the baby was born, students were expected to visit each day while the mother and infant were in the hospital. In 1952, staff patients were hospitalized four days with a first baby, and three days with a subsequent baby. If the baby was born by cesarean, the mother and baby would be hospitalized 7 to 10 days. It was clear, as Dr. Kennell observed the interactions between students and mothers, that these post-delivery visits became very important to both mothers and students; a special, yet "mysterious" relationship developed.

After the baby was discharged to home, students were expected not only to make home visits, but also to attend visits of the baby to pediatric clinics that were scattered around Cleveland. However, the planners of the program had not anticipated how widely dispersed these clinics could be. In addition, mothers would be given an appointment time, but would often have to wait several hours, along with the students, before the physician was available.

Finally, the clinic experience was not particularly educational because the physicians were very busy and took little time to explain things to the students. It became clear that the original plan did not provide an effective learning situation for students. Therefore, a decision was made to arrange for well-baby visits at Babies and Children's Hospital Out Patient Department. This program became known as the Family Clinic, and John Kennell was asked to direct it. Initially, the space provided had little privacy, but eventually there was general recognition about who could use the examining rooms in the Family Clinic area.

Dr. Kennell noted that families assigned to the medical students included both mother and father, although, only some were married. Some families already had several children. Many of the mothers were adolescents. The program elected not to include mothers who were less than 15 years old. Dr. Kennell was the only pediatric instructor in the Family Clinic during its first year. Later, other pediatricians from the Cleveland community participated as volunteers.

Giving Students More Responsibility

Dr. Kennell stated:

> The medical students were very excited about coming to that first clinic visit. They paid close attention to everything I said and the mother said … They often would have observations that were very helpful about what the home was like, and who was there, and what was going on.

However, by the second or third visit, it was apparent that the students were not as interested in what the mother said, or what Dr. Kennelll said. Unfortunately, faculty had made the decision that students would have no responsibility to take histories, examine the infant, and then present their findings to the family clinic faculty. The suggestion that the students should be given more responsibility was met by a "firm negative response."

As one might expect, Dr. Kennell persisted in his determination to give students more responsibility. Eventually, both Dr. Wallace, the Chair of Pediatrics, and Dr. Spector supported him at faculty meetings. The decision was made that students could take more responsibility by taking the history of the babies whom they were following, but not do the infant physical exams. As a compromise, Dr. Kennell would invite students to watch a faculty member do a certain part of the physical exam, and then would allow them to repeat that exam. Over the course of a year, each student would gain experience in doing each part of the examination. After several years, students were allowed to do the entire examination with faculty supervision. Because the clinic became busier and more crowded, Dr. Kennell started the practice of having students go to the home of the infant prior to the scheduled appointment to update the history and to make observations in the home.

Dr. Spock and Justifying the Program

The Family Clinic was part of what attracted Dr. Spock to Cleveland. Dr. Kennell has related:

> Douglas Bond was head of psychiatry and a very excellent salesperson ... He started to persuade Dr. Ben Spock to come to Cleveland ... Lo and behold he came in 1955 ... I was in great awe of him and although I never took a course from him, I learned a great deal by working with him in the pediatric Family Clinic ... He was a big man, confident, and very likable. I think he came at a time very important to the Family Clinic, and me, because he had stature, and a lot of people thought it was kind of crazy to have a student program like that.

Dr. Kennell has also asserted that Dr. Spock's famous 1946 book, *Baby and Child Care*, earned him only 5 cents a copy! By participating in Dr. Spock's "Child Rearing Study," which lasted at least 35 years, there were many additional opportunities for Dr. Kennell to discuss patient issues.

Each year in the 1950s, the Dean of the Western Reserve Medical School, Dr. Joseph Wearn, held a meeting at a schoolhouse in Gates Mills for faculty to review the medical education program. There were vigorous debates in this forum, including those about the Family Clinic, which was regarded as strange and unusual. For Dr. Kennell, it was stressful to prepare a report each year. There would be questions about all sorts of things in the program.

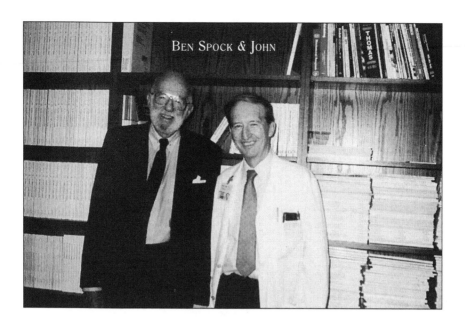

BEN SPOCK & JOHN

New faculty, who had not previously heard about it, would have new objections. Afterwards, some supporters would say, "Boy, they really battered you, didn't they? I felt really sorry for you." Yet, the enthusiasm of the clinical faculty and students kept the Family Clinic going. He remained as director until 1960, when he took on a position at the Green Road Rainbow Hospital.

Eventually, Dr. Kennell accumulated data about the numbers of students, their attendance, and the benefits to them, and published a long 1961 article in *The Journal of Medical Education*. It included eight sections that described the general plan, personnel and facilities, student experience and learning, family attitudes, and analyses of responses of families and physicians in training. Later objections to the program were stilled when it became very clear that many good students enrolled in the medical school on account of the program. Students were very proud of what they were doing.

Program Modifications

Dr. Kennell was always interested in improving communication and learning among all participants in his world. Therefore, as part of the Family Clinic program, he organized groups of 6-to-10 first-year medical students to review family needs with a social worker and a pediatrician. The social workers and pediatricians found this very helpful, although, occasionally there were students who were uninterested in babies and children. Beginning students faced many challenges. Preceptors helped by emphasizing to parents that the services of the student were valuable, and would point out how well the student did in examining a certain part of the baby (e.g., the heart).

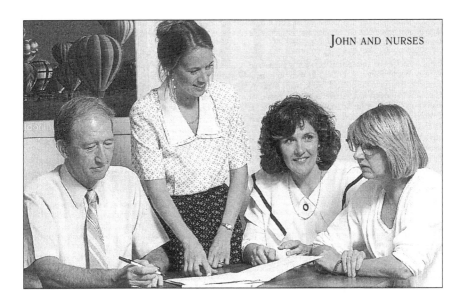

JOHN AND NURSES

Sometimes a mother was shy, and students would have difficulty obtaining information about the baby. Students would be dismayed when mothers would reveal pertinent elements of the history to the pediatrician that they had not mentioned to the students. Dr. Kennell told how:

> It was a delicate matter to support the student and teach the student without criticizing in any kind of threatening or harmful way. Once students became more confident, the mother began to appreciate that she had a doctor who was learning and doing the same things that regular doctors did.

There were also efforts to provide a central telephone number for messages for mothers, students, and faculty.

During the early years of the program, medical students followed the infants for the entire four years of medical school. During the third year of medical school, they were assigned an adult patient. If possible, arrangements were made for the adult patients to be the father or mother of the infant whom they had been following for the previous two years. Medical students examined their adult patients in a clinic in the Internal Medicine Department.

Over time, there were further changes in the medical school curriculum, and the numbers of medical students increased from 82 to 150. Students who were at a different location in their third-year clerkships were in the awkward position of being unable to see their families in the Family Clinic when they had a new patient in their clerkship. Still, the student could discuss the problem of the family with the Family Clinic preceptor, in spite of an inability to actually see the patient. In the fourth year, the clinical responsibilities of students became yet more complex.

Consequently, in the 1980s, a decision was made to have students follow the families only during their first two years in medical school. At this point, there would be a painful separation, for both families and students. Dr. Kennell remarked:

> The families didn't understand it, and while some medical students were happy to be free of the responsibility, most were sad to leave. We had several experiences where students did not follow those rules, and kept in touch with the mothers. They might go to the emergency room when the child became sick. We had situations in which students were not being supervised ... and continuing as the doctor, even though they weren't the doctor. Medical students cannot prescribe, not having a license. They were not in a legal position to function as a physician. So we had to

establish guidelines about how the student could stay in touch with the family legally.

Faculty members discussed the problem of termination with families at their meetings, and did their best to help students with this stress. Some students begged to stay on with their assigned families. For some, the faculty would agree that they could stop by the Family Clinic from time to time to say hello to their families. Dr. Kennell observed over 50 years that returning alumni of the medical school were generally most interested in finding out how their family was doing. This continued as the babies they followed reached adulthood. Some followed their families by letter and others by phone. As years passed, younger students would contact students in senior classes to get advice about the program. They also gained help and insight from the preceptor groups.

The program sadly folded in 2006 for financial reasons.

Clinical Sciences

The Clinical Science Program for medical students was also part of the 1951 Western Reserve Medical School curriculum revision. For many years, the Family Clinic was a large component of the Clinical Science Program because patients who were discussed in the Clinical Science preceptor groups came from the Family Clinic.

Dr. Kennell was a preceptor for the Clinical Science groups for more than 50 years. The groups, as originally defined, had two preceptors. One was a faculty member, and the other was a social worker or someone who had experience with pediatrics in the community.

The groups would attend a lecture together, or visit a hospitalized patient, and the meeting would conclude with discussion and wrap-up. Students had opportunities to visit other institutions in the community, including hospitals, homes for the elderly, and facilities for handicapped individuals. Early on, during the first year of medical school, there was a training session on children born with malformations and handicaps, such as Down syndrome. Students would have the opportunity to talk with parents of a child with handicaps, and to learn about their many challenges. Faculty would provide background reading material for the students. All students in a group gradually knew about all the families, followed by other members of the group.

During the first two or three years of the Clinical Science program, meetings largely focused on helping the student in the group who had most recently been assigned a family. Everyone wanted to hear every detail about the labor and delivery. Other students asked many questions. Preceptors sought to provide enough time for each student to present their whole family and tell their experiences in meeting the patient at home, in the clinic and then during labor and delivery.

During the group meetings, priority was given to families with special developments, such as having a baby who had been discharged, then developed a fever and returned to the hospital. It was hoped that all the students would learn from these special situations and the follow-up recommendations. During the first 25 years of the program, students were told to call a preceptor if there was a medical problem in the family. Often, these problems involved an illness in one of the parents. Students also were asked to sign out to someone else during holidays, such as Thanksgiving, Christmas, or summer break, and to inform the mother about arrangements.

Dr. Kennell commented about the preceptors for the program:

> When I first started, a variety of physicians were the preceptors and not every doctor is wild about pediatrics and children and pregnant women ... During the first 10 years the Department of Pediatrics provided several pediatric preceptors. Some continued for a year and some longer. As the demands of hospital care increased, it was difficult for many physicians to serve as preceptors for more than one year.

There were some community pediatricians who were faithful preceptors for many years. Examples included Dr. Mary Hellerstein, Dr. Israel Weisberg, and Dr. Irving Weintraub. The Chair of Obstetrics provided two obstetricians each year for the first 10 years of the program. One would be a full-time faculty obstetrician, and one would be a community obstetrician. Eventually, a special obstetrics clinic was established to care for the mothers, and to teach students during the pregnancy phase of the Family Clinic Program.

As the family clinic program progressed, new issues arose. Students would make long visits to the family, and would be offered meals or participation in family social activities. Kennell and colleagues told students that although it was good to be friendly and play with children for a while, it was also important to recognize the professional aspects of their student responsibilities.

Another issue related to the fact that students often had cars, and families did not. Some students offered to pick up families or drive them home. Kennell's group decided that this could be done only in an emergency. When the program began, there were no emergency services for transport to the hospital. As professional emergency transportation became available, and a "provide a ride" service was established for clinic visits, the practice of student-provided transport was discouraged because of legal implications.

There were visitors to the Family Clinic. A professor from India visited and set up a similar clinic in his medical school in India, although he had only one full-time faculty member to help him. When Kennell asked him how he could succeed with so little help, the Indian professor said, "One must do this. Our medical students come from all over India, but they have no idea how people live in the area around our hospital."

That was also true for the majority of medical students in the CWRU Family Clinic. Kennell speculated that the Family Clinic experience impacted life choices of some of the medical students.

Dr. Kennell stated that a "marvelous group" started the first (1951) curriculum revision at Western Reserve Medical School. Some faculty continued to precept medical student groups in the Clinical Science (later called Fundamentals of Clinical Practice) program for more than 40 years. As time went on, hospitals were less willing to release staff, such as nurses, to participate in the groups. Group leaders sought retired health care professionals, including social workers and community nurses.

Over the years, when the follow-up period was reduced from four to two years, many groups took increasing lengths of time to acquire their full group of families. Kennell noted that medical care and systems were changing, and the social environment had also changed. In the beginning, each infant had an involved father and mother.

As years passed, most families included a mother and infant only. Mothers would sign up for one medical insurance program in one location, and then changes led to her being assigned to medical services farther away. Some mothers found the longer distances and multiple bus changes too complicated. Families were more transient and mobile. So fewer families were available, and many medical students did not have a new baby to follow until towards the end of their first year.

The changes led to changing processes within the groups. Relevant topics were assigned to all groups. For example, if families had children with developmental or behavioral problems, these topics would be assigned to all students in the group. One or two of the students would be asked to present and discuss what they had found in the literature. There were many opportunities to facilitate group discussion on a range of pediatric topics. This was especially important for the students who were following babies in their second year of life, but who were no longer seeing the family as often. Preceptors made efforts to teach about the relationship between what happens—or doesn't happen—in the second year of life, and effects on the third and fourth year of life.

Dr. Kennell continued to precept in the Clinical Science program long after he was no longer working in the Family Clinic. Increasingly, his hearing limitations became a problem in the medical-student groups. He said:

> During my last five years as a group preceptor, my hearing was getting worse and the co-preceptor was Kathy Cole Kelly. She was an excellent leader and really too trained to be a co-preceptor. I had to take second place and often did not know exactly what the topic was ... I learned that it's difficult for students to appreciate a handicap, so before I would start the year I would explain I couldn't hear very well, and would ask that students speak up and try to look directly at me. It's very quickly forgotten ... When students began to come with laptops, they would have their laptop open and looking at it during their presentation ... I would request that it would be nice if the students who weren't presenting something could look up at me ... I had all sorts of hearing aids, but you get to the point where they aren't adequate so that's when you have to quit.

Several pediatricians who directed the Family Clinic succeeded Dr. Kennell. The most recent directors were Dr. Fred Heggie (1995 to 2000) and Dr. Mireille Boutry, who was director until 2005. The program ended because of the combination of recruitment difficulties and the belief of the medical school dean that medical students would benefit more from seeing a variety of short-term patients rather than continuity with a few families. Drs. Mary Hellerstein and Arthur Burns remained with the program the entire time.

Note: John Kennell quotations were taken from unpublished interviews conducted by Mary Hellerstein, MD on March 21, 2007 and August 30, 2007.

Chapter 5
RAINBOW ON GREEN ROAD

Evolution of a Hospital

D r. Kennell had become very devoted to the Family Clinic, so it was a difficult separation for him when he was assigned his next responsibility at Rainbow Hospital for Children. Between 1961 and 1965, he was the Pediatrician-in-Charge there. He explains,

> The Hospital was on Green Road, in a lovely English-type setting with long grass fields . . . By 1960, it was a children's hospital for rehabilitation and long-term care . . . My duties were quite different, but they fit with some of my pediatric training. I had a couple months at the house of the Good Samaritan in Boston, which was affiliated with Children's Hospital. It had been a center of research on how to care for children with rheumatic fever.

There, Dr. Kennell was able to learn much from the faculty member who had done most of the studies.

Dr. Kennell was a firm supporter of Rainbow and its Board of Directors. The book, *For the Children*, describes its history (Horwitz et al., 2007). The hospital began on Thanksgiving Day, 1887, when nine young women, all friends, came together to discuss how they could help poor children in the Cleveland area. Most were still teenagers, and they all came from prominent, wealthy, industrial, and commercial families in Cleveland. They called themselves, "Rainbow Circle of King's Daughters," part of an international volunteer movement of young women volunteers. These women, their families, and many other families who joined them, sought to provide a supportive environment for children to recover from an illness, such as tuberculosis or rheumatic fever. They first established Rainbow Cottage in 1891, in what is now Bratenahl. Following several other care facilities, and an expanding circle of supporters, a new Rainbow Hospital for Crippled and Convalescent Children opened on Green Road in 1905. By 1928, it was part of the University Hospital System, including the Western Reserve School of Medicine, and was housed in a new single floor building on Green Road. The mission of long-term rehabilitation, with an emphasis on orthopedics, never changed, and it continued to add supportive activities.

The Child Life Connection

Dr. Kennell stated:

> It had been busier in previous times . . . Minimal visiting by parents was allowed. I met Thesi Bergman at Rainbow Hospital. She was a very warm, thoughtful, patient woman who did her best to help the children at Rainbow, providing toys and reading material. However, she was one person and there were 50 children, so her ability to provide individualized attention was limited.

You could say this was the beginning of Child Life for Babies and Children's. Thesi Bergman was a psychologist and former colleague of Anna Freud, and had been at Rainbow over a decade. Dr. Kennell continued:

> When I was there I focused on research studies related to rheumatic fever, and sometimes on polio, when there would

be big epidemics and most of the hospitalized children were recovering from polio. What I observed during the polio epidemic caused me great consternation. The children were in a long ward, and told never to walk, and never to step out of bed. There was an iron pipe that held up the curtain, so this one little fellow swung on it as far as he could possibly go. The nurses caught him. There was a big uproar about that.

Once again Dr. Kennell could see a need for change:

There was beginning to be more and more interest in changing policy about bed rest since there was increasing evidence that bed rest was not a helpful treatment for many conditions . . . Obviously, children who were in congestive heart failure, and children on the verge of congestive heart failure, had to be in bed, but there were others who were doing quite well. Gradually we had courage to allow more children to be active while in the hospital, although we followed them nervously at first.

Rainbow had served many hospitals, but in 1971, Babies and Children's and Rainbow merged hospitals both in name and physically (see chapter 8). The new Rainbow Babies and Children's Hospital (RB&C) included one specific Rainbow Division that accommodated the orthopedists associated with Rainbow. There they could admit patients, perform surgeries, and follow the recovery of their patients in one place.

Note: John Kennell quotations were taken from an unpublished interview conducted by Mary Hellerstein, MD on August 23, 2007.

Chapter 6
SABBATICAL IN ENGLAND

A Year with the Family

By 1965, Dr. Kennell began to appreciate the need for more training, particularly in psychiatry, even though he "wasn't wild about psycho-analysis." He had the opportunity to take a sabbatical from his duties at Rainbow Hospital in 1966 to 1967. The idea of expanding his geographical horizons was also appealing.

Dr. Kennell recalled that this was an important year for the family "because [they] were strangers, [they] did a lot of things together." The schools, the underground, sports, miniskirts—everything was new for them. While the family's experiences might be new, Dr. Kennell noted:

> Everything in England was old . . . It was 20 years after the war and in the United States we had forgotten about it, but it was evident everywhere. Everything was backward and limited . . . People lived very frugally because of the war.

Dr. Kennell's shoes would wear out quickly from walking across the heath, but he was told he must replace them with English shoes. Nothing else could tolerate the constant wet. A break in the English weather, even less sunny than Cleveland, might cheerfully be reported as "bright periods" with a "little more light" than usual. Meager background heating in their home left the family cold the entire time. It definitely helped to have a lovely spring, which came with flowering trees and beautiful flowers that would last a long time.

An English school classmate and friend of Dr. Kennell's, Kenneth Holt, had just moved from the northern part of England. He helped the Kennell family get settled only two blocks from his own home. Since both families were new arrivals, they enjoyed exploring the city together. Following World War II, Dr. Holt had become known for his neurological observations about children with handicaps. Ultimately, he became the head of the Department of Developmental Paediatrics at the University of London.

Dr. Kennell's plan for a fellowship in child psychology may not have materialized, but these were inspirational days for him. What he learned confirmed what his 20 years of experience had shown him; that traditional visitation rules in children's hospitals were devastating for the children. He learned much from James Robertson and Anna Freud.

James Robertson and "A Two-Year-Old Goes to Hospital"

Dr. Kennell described the life of James Robertson as follows:

> James Robertson was born in a large, very poor family in Scotland. I may be wrong, but something like seven children would sleep in a bed. It's hard to imagine. When World War II began, there was great pressure to get everybody into the service. James Robertson was a conscientious objector, and he was given several tasks. One somehow got him involved with children, primarily from London, who were (removed from their families) and taken to an area where it was thought to be safer than right in the heart of London. So he was exposed to a lot of children who must have been under great distress away from their family. It's

easy to criticize . . . but if you think of the mighty German air force and its almost unrestricted bombing of England at the beginning of the war, you can see why parents and doctors and others thought getting (the children) out of the city would be the safest thing to do. Families and children were not prepared for that.

James Robertson developed a great interest in children, subsequently becoming a psychoanalyst and psychiatric social worker. His wife, Joyce Robertson, "a marvelous, bright woman," obtained training at the Anna Freud Wartime Nurseries. Dr. Kennell continues:

James Robertson also developed skills in film making, and made a film that had enormous impact. It's hard to think of anything in pediatrics that had quite such a large impact, particularly in England and the United States in psychological circles . . . That (1952 film) was called, *A Two Year Old Goes to Hospital,* and I do recommend it to all people going into pediatrics. That film was shocking, and it was shown to pediatricians first. They had terribly negative reactions . . . There was one pediatrician whom I met in England, Dermod MacCarthy . . . He was wildly upset. I think he was awake all night. Then during the night he began to think about it. A few days later he talked to James Robertson and said, "I do things differently with my patients at the hospital I'm connected with. Why don't you come and film a mother and her baby there?"

Robertson then made a second film that came out in 1958: the name was, *Going to Hospital with Mother.* When I was in England, I went to his hospital, and went to the room where that occurred. I saw there a mother with a young child just as in the movie.

Dr. Kennell felt that if anyone had seen the two films in juxtaposition, it would be easy to determine which approach was best.

> In the second film, the mother stayed with the child . . . fed the child, and diapered the child, and took general care of the youngster. Children with a variety of conditions sailed through hospitalization very smoothly, in marked contrast to those without mothers present. The one who went to the hospital without her mother (in the first film) was a determined young lady who held up and fought against things quite well, at first. Then she got very upset and very angry. Because they followed that child for a long time, they saw remnants of that experience that would keep popping up later on. James Robertson was working with Dr. John Bowlby, and it fit in well with what Dr. Bowlby was finding out in his psychoanalytic observations.

> By the time I was in England, there was certainly a beginning appreciation of these findings. I didn't hear criticism from many pediatricians about mothers going to the hospital with their babies.

Anna Freud

Dr. Kennell would meet many outstanding doctors and investigators, some involved in international child health. Anna Freud was a huge attraction for students and professionals. Even though Dr. Kennell really did not have the appropriate training, he persisted in attending whatever meetings he could that were mentored by Anna Freud. There were very lively exchanges, where everyone learned. He came to appreciate her more and more, and would approach her later as a person who was also deeply interested in children. She had "a warm way about her," and was respectful of doctors, but very forthright. He was astonished by an exchange he had the last time he saw Anna Freud.

She said, "Oh, Dr. Kennell, I have an important question for you. Are all babies the same at birth?" I said, "No, no, no, they are different as can be." She said she went through a long list of American psychoanalysts that come (to England) and 'they all tell me the babies are the same at birth.' I said, "They are so different—and Barry Brazelton did a lot of studies showing how different babies respond—and there are very important differences." Anna Freud said, "I always thought so."

Notes: Quotations are taken from a series of interviews with John Kennell conducted by Mary Hellerstein, MD between March and August 2007.

Chapter 7

BEREAVEMENT GROUPS FOR PARENTS WHO HAD LOST YOUNG CHILDREN

D r. Kennell often talked about the grief he personally felt when children died. When he was a young house officer, many more hospitalized children died than is true today. As director of the premature nursery at Babies and Children's Hospital, he witnessed the death of many infants. One reason was respiratory distress. The most common treatment was provision of oxygen, and it sometimes led to retrolental fibroplasias (damage to the retina), which caused blindness in survivors.

At one point, Dr. Kennell organized an early, unpublished trial showing that a reduced oxygen level would produce fewer side effects. Unfortunately, oxygen treatment did not address the basic problem, which was a deficiency in lung surfactant.

The importance of surfactant in facilitating newborn respiration was not understood at that time. Surfactant was isolated only in 1961, by his future collaborator, Dr. Marshall Klaus, who went on to test it along with other investigators.

Although, doctors and nurses worked hard to take care of critically ill premature infants, there was little sensitivity to the grief parents experienced when their premature children died. Dr. Kennell described the treatment of bodies of deceased prematures as follows:

> At that time in the medical school, we had a revision of the curriculum. As part of the revision, there was discussion about the fact that many premature babies died, and families were given the opportunity to have the baby's body taken care of by the hospital, without charge to the family. Because the new curriculum included a program that allowed medical students to follow a pregnant woman in the obstetric clinic, remain with the mother during labor and delivery, and to visit the mother and infant in the days

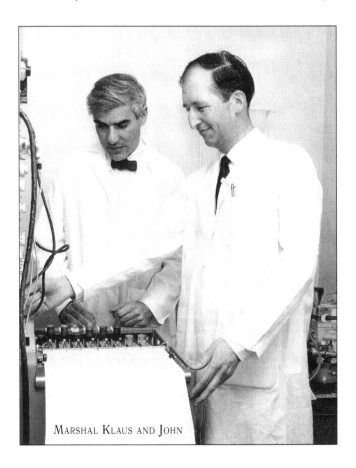

MARSHAL KLAUS AND JOHN

following birth, it was proposed that the bodies of infants signed over to the hospital for disposition would be used for dissection by the medical students. That plan was approved. Each cadaver was used by a group of several students, giving them an introduction to the anatomy of a newborn.

A Medical-Student-Inspired Study

Shortly after Dr. Kennell returned from sabbatical, and began working with Dr. Klaus in the late 1960s, a medical student, Howard Slyter, came to them and said he was interested in the death of newborns and reactions to that death. The resulting randomized study led to a special article (Kennell et al. 1970). Dr. Kennell said,

> This was again a lesson to me. It's awfully easy to get focused so solidly on one issue, or one patient, that you don't appreciate all their difficulties. We certainly were aware that the loss of a premature baby was a very important loss to families, but it became shockingly apparent from this research. We had a series of questions to find out about events that went on during the death of the baby and afterwards.

The team proceeded to contact families who had lost premature infants. While it was difficult to ask the questions, some families were willing to participate, despite the depth of their grief. Because of the rules about parent visitation, the mothers might or might not have seen the baby prior to death. Even if the babies lived a little while, and the mother may have seen or touched the baby, most of the deaths occurred very soon after birth. At that time, no one thought to give the mother pictures, or clothing, or locks of hair as mementoes of their babies.

Due to this kind of information from bereaved parents, Dr. Kennell and his colleagues were led to examine the writings of Dr. Erich Lindemann, who was a psychiatrist in Boston at the time of the Coconut Grove fire. A large number of young, healthy sailors, soldiers, and marines were celebrating before they embarked for Europe or the Pacific. The fire spread rapidly. Doors opened easily from the outside, but not from the inside, and close to 500 people died in the fire. Lindeman went to homes to interview the bereaved families. He recognized a series of stages that were shown by the majority of parents of the young adults who died. Their mourning was intense and went on for a very long time. The parents never got over it.

Dr. Kennell and colleagues found similarities between those reactions and those of mothers who had lost a newborn. The mothers had all sorts of dreams and expectations for their child, but they didn't have an opportunity to know their child. They had perceived the infant inside them, and may have had a glimpse of the infant at the time of delivery or in an incubator. That was all. Their reactions were severe. For all of us who have never had or seen a preterm baby, the thought of looking at one's own baby and perceiving it as an animal is completely incomprehensible. It was striking for Dr. Kennell and his colleagues to learn that about half of the mothers and fathers having terrible reactions had not talked about the baby a single time after they left the hospital. This was in contrast to mothers who had spent time with their baby or older child prior to death; all they could think about or talk about was their child.

Death, an Ignored Subject

The parents who had lost a premature infant had no basis for discussion. With no effort made to help parents talk to each other during the birth and hospitalization, they just couldn't talk about the death. It was too upsetting. Dr. Lindemann and many others have written about this topic and emphasized the importance of talking about the baby, the death, the feelings, and talking with other people who have had a loss. Dr. Kennell and colleagues recognized that the parents of most premature infants in the United States were not given that opportunity. This was shocking to Dr. Kennell and his group. He decided to do something about it.

The group realized that there had been nothing written about the death of a child in popular literature since the book, *Little Women*. In that story, Beth died of scarlet fever. That appeared to be the last time that the death of a child was mentioned in a novel for the lay public.

Dr. Kennell initiated changes in how families were treated after the death of a newborn. Every effort was made to provide a quiet room where the mother, father, and family members, including other children, could stay together for as long as they wished. They might close the door and ask not to be disturbed, but a staff person would be available and attentive to their needs. Medical staff, including physicians and nurses, had meetings to consider how to help the bereaved families. For example, families might treasure a cap that was on the infant, a lock of hair, an item of clothing, or even fingerprints of the baby. Most obstetrical units in the United States are now similarly helpful to families who lose an infant at the time of birth.

Although nurses are attentive to the needs of parents at the time of an infant's death, if the infant has been in the nursery very briefly, there may have been no nurse with a connection to that infant or family. Dr. Kennell observed that even when the infant had been hospitalized a long time, and the nurses knew the family well, it was still difficult for many nurses to call the family to see how they were doing.

This topic has been beautifully discussed in the chapter, "Coping with a Stillborn or an Infant Who Dies," in *Bonding: The Beginnings of Parent-Infant Attachment,* by Drs. Klaus and Kennell. Mothers reported feeling that they had created death, failed as women, or were left with an unbearable emptiness. Hoping to spare the parents, physicians would keep them away from the baby, not realizing that most parents needed to experience the reality of the death, for proof of the baby's existence. One woman was offered a tranquilizer when she started to cry. Most important was providing reassurance that the baby would never be forgotten and could never be replaced. The authors recommended having at least three visits with parents: an immediate meeting to describe that there's a normal mourning process; one at 2 to 3 days to listen a lot and to review reactions that can occur during grieving; and one at 3 to 6 months to verify that healthy, rather than pathological, grieving is taking place.

Development of Grief Groups

Dr. Kennell thought it likely that some of the bereaved parents would benefit if they could get together with other parents who had also lost an infant in the premature nursery. Therefore, when two bereaved couples approached the investigators about having a parents' group, they organized a group in 1971. This was called Parents Experiencing a Neonatal Death (PEND). It would meet once a month for 3 hours in the evening. Ultimately, parents attended from the whole area of greater Cleveland, and from several distant areas.

Drs. Kennell and Klaus asked two bereaved couples to lead the first group. Both doctors tried to say as little as possible, but to allow the bereaved parents to speak. Discussions were honest, including occasional criticisms of the actions of the doctors themselves. These groups were greatly appreciated by the families and, because of the demand, the size of the meeting room had to be increased. However, when parents had been coming to the group for several months, and had become quite well acquainted, they might begin to talk about issues of little emotional significance. At the same time, more recently bereaved parents were struggling; many parents were unable to speak at their first group meeting. Still, the support of the group would enable them to share their feelings in subsequent meetings. At one point, there were so many parents that Dr. Kennell suggested to those who had been coming for a long time that they might skip a meeting or two so there would be more time to focus on the recently bereaved. Those parents said, "You can't do that to us, Dr. Kennell, we need this."

Dr. Kennell noted that women who were pregnant with a subsequent pregnancy, especially, needed to continue group support. He also found that female parent leaders were the most effective. Lengthy phone discussions between group participants and parent leaders sometimes took place between meetings, and could be very helpful.

After managed care was introduced in the Cleveland community, each hospital stated that it was providing many services, including bereavement groups. Consequently, attendance at PEND groups at Rainbow Babies and Children's Hospital decreased. Except when he was out of Cleveland, Dr. Kennell attended every meeting of the PEND group for 35 years, until 2006. It is, of course, doubtful that every hospital could have a person as dedicated as Dr. Kennell to organize, and stay with, the bereavement groups for parents. Dr. Kennell stated,

> This is a reminder of the unpleasantness to everybody of dealing with death. The fact is that it is much more stimulating and rewarding to work with the living and help a baby recover from a bad situation . . . There continue to be many families that appear to be just like the families that so appreciated PEND. It's difficult not to believe there are still many parents in our community who need this opportunity and are not obtaining it.

Dr. Kennell always worried about whether someone would continue these groups.

Note: John Kennell quotations were taken from an unpublished interview conducted by Mary Hellerstein, MD on June 13, 2007.

Chapter 8
CHILD LIFE AND THE
NEW HOSPITAL

C hild Life, as it developed into the professional, credentialed system of services that it is today, did not bloom instantly. The necessity for caring for the needs of the child and their families beyond treating the child's illness took time to establish. In Cleveland, psychiatry played a formative role. Emma Planck had trained with Montessori in Rome, studied with Sigmund and Anna Freud in Vienna, and left Europe in the face of WWII. She passed through California on her way to Cleveland in 1951 to direct the Therapeutic Nursery School at University Hospitals. Dr. Fredrick Robbins, who was the head of the Department of Pediatrics at the Hospital that is now Metro Health, recruited her in 1955. He wanted her to focus on the needs of children requiring extended care, such as those with TB (drugs were not yet widely available).

Emma Planck founded the Child Life program at Metro Health Medical Center. Dr. Kennell reported that she was also the leader of Child Life programs at Mt. Sinai Hospital, and that they were envious of her programs at Babies and Children's Hospital. Leaders at Rainbow and Green Road would attend most of Emma Planck's meetings related to child life activities and make good presentations. The Child Life program supported individual nurses and others who, for a long time, wanted to make the hospital environment more home-like for families. He could see how happy the nursing staff members were with the program, and how eager they were to support it. He noted that families and children are indebted to the many people who had pioneering ideas back in the early part of the 20th century, regarding the treatment of hospitalized children, and who did studies, such as those of James Robertson.

The chairman of pediatrics from 1952 to 1968, Dr. William Wallace "was a marvelous man, who was very sound in all regards," affirmed Dr. Kennell. When he first came to Cleveland, parent visiting was allowed once a week, for half an hour on Saturday afternoons. When Anna Freud came in 1952, Dr. Wallace asked her what she thought about visiting hours. She said she thought mothers ought to be with their children whenever they wanted. According to Marshall Klaus (2000), a resident at the time,

> She spoke on hospitalization, and the significance of hospitalization, on a Friday. The next Monday, Bill Wallace changed the hospital rules and there was visiting every day.

As Dr. Kennell noted,

> Changes don't occur smoothly overnight, so there were often restrictions about not coming until mid-morning, so the doctors and nurses could do their activities. But, in general, and obviously if it was a very sick child or critically ill child, the parent would be allowed to stay.

Dr. Kennell was always appreciative of the wisdom of mothers. He found in the clinic that:

> [E]xperienced mothers, black or white, would be tremendously helpful if there was a formal or informal group discussion . . . They would come in with a suggestion that would be helpful to me and reassuring to the mother.

Play Ladies Evolve into Child Life Specialists

Dr. Kennell stated,

> When I first came to Babies and Children's Hospital in 1952, I don't remember any planned system for providing play activities for children. I think they were kept in their beds, as they were in Boston. Studies were underway when I left Boston that showed clearly there was a great advantage to have women who came and helped with the children...I remember a wonderfully warm woman who was at the admitting desk at Babies and Children's Hospital . . . If a child was going to be admitted, the family was directed into an admitting area, where she took the telephone calls and guided people around. I hardly remember seeing her when she didn't have a baby or young child she was looking after. She could do a lot with a baby in one arm. I think her example led to the conversion of an adjoining area into a play area. Toys were very limited, and crude, and no fun, but there were some very creative people. I have a letter from a former worker at that play area telling how cleverly she developed all sorts of toys out of simple objects. It's a reminder that it doesn't take a lot of money and fancy electronic toys to make children happy. The women who did that were called play ladies and assistants, and a good many were volunteers. Many had been at Rainbow Hospital.

Child Life at Babies and Children's became official when Jennie Lyons was hired as the first salaried play lady in 1959.

During that time, from the mid-1950s to 1970s, there were a number of favorable influences that contributed to the development of Child Life programs. The Department of Child Psychiatry at University Hospitals of Cleveland had a number of women who had trained as child therapists with Anna Freud.

They were involved with some patients in Babies and Children's Hospital, but most of their activities were at the Hanna Perkins Center, which opened in 1961. Cleveland also benefited from Anna Freud's many visits. She was highly respected, and shared her knowledge with both medical students and professionals. Dr. Klaus noted that this profoundly wise woman never dressed formally, but rather, like a grandmother.

By the late 60s, there were more divisional therapists—more play therapists and more play ladies. Their title now shifted to Child Life Worker. In 1969, a director of Child Life activities, Edward Gratzick, was chosen. Dr. Kennell continued:

> Not to downplay anything about the abilities of women, but at that time I think it was a very opportune selection. I think it was easier for him to fit in with the male physicians at meal times and at some meetings, and I think he carried a little more weight with the administrative people. He was there five years. When he left there was a succession of very fine women.

As time went on, Child Life took on many roles, becoming more professional. Later, staff members would be called Child Life Specialists and, along with other duties, would help children and their parents prepare for procedures.

Rooming In and the New Hospital

While Child Life was gaining momentum, plans for the new hospital were being made. As Dr. Kennell elaborated,

> Dr. Scott Dowling was a child psychiatrist who was doing studies at Babies and Children's Hospital, so he was well known and appreciated by the staff, medical, nursing, and other staff. We both felt it was very important at this time to apply what had been shown in England. By that time, it

had been shown in a couple other hospitals. There was one in Boston that had a special unit where they had a big genitourinary program. They had quite a large area that was for the children admitted for those studies and they allowed mothers to stay. We went and observed it and did our best to promote facilities for all mothers to live in with their babies.

However, this was such a foreign concept, that others were not easily convinced. Dr. Kennell further elaborated:

> Dr. Wallace was a scientist so he was very careful about things and he checked with the heads of pediatrics at the major centers and then told me, "A lot of them said it was crazy to provide that space. The mothers wouldn't come. Some estimated 20% of mothers might come, but it wouldn't be much more than that." The number that he was able to sell to other people was 20%."

Although, it was only 20% of rooms, in the history account, *For the Children*, it is stated that the new hospital was "a milestone in the evolution of family-centered care, thanks to the advocacy and efforts of many professionals, most notably John Kennell and Dalia Zemaitye."

It took several years to physically build the new hospital. Following an amazing plan beginning in July of 1969, the old hospital was jacked up, put on railroad tracks and moved 80 feet, so part of the new hospital could be built in its space. One can only imagine the stress accompanying the logistics of temporarily moving patients into the adult hospital, tending to anxious parents, and filling staffing requirements for patients who could not be sent home.

However, that was just the beginning. Within a month, the utilities in the old building were reconnected and continued to serve patients and their families. No major problems occurred. The new hospital was ready in September of 1971.

Dr. Kennell explained,

> It was really exciting the first day that it was open. There
> were a number of people who had heard about it somehow.
> There was great demand for the 20% . . . designed to have
> an adult bed for the mother and a crib for the baby or child.
> The first few days we made out. Then in the first week a
> doctor who had referred me a number of patients in the
> past called and said, "John, I hate to bother you with this. I
> know you are busy but I have this patient that came in last
> night and she has a little pneumonia, and we are going to
> be able to take care of her just fine, but her mother has
> heard about your unit and she is insisting she's going to take
> the baby out if we don't arrange for her to go to a hospital
> where she can stay with the child."

Such calls continued, so the hospital found it necessary to convert
the rooms designed for mother and child, to rooms with two cribs and then
somehow make do for the mothers. At first, a mother would have an ordinary
chair, then a softer chair, and eventually a reclining chair, or even a cot. In
general, it was not great sleeping.

Because of the popularity of allowing mothers to stay with their children,
each floor was reconstructed to provide a room where the mother could sit
during the day and meet with other mothers. Equipped with toilet facilities and
a shower, the arrangement changed an inadequate situation into a reasonably
good one. The rooms also became important for discussing private or serious
matters with families. Dr. Kennell continued,

> Rooming in was such a successful venture that every hospital
> in Cleveland soon provided that. The spirit and behavior
> of everybody on the division was different because you
> knew all the time there were parents present. Parents were
> anxious, of course. They would interrupt nurses, but they

would do all sorts of things to help other mothers, or tell nurses about problems, or help feed a baby if something came up that took the mother away. With the success of rooming in, we had everything in place for a very fine Child Life program. I'm pleased to say that program was really magic for our hospital.

With regard to premature babies, as time went along and the science continued to improve, not only did more tiny babies live, but also the involvement of families was maintained. A step-down unit in a new 1985 hospital addition was provided for mothers to stay with their sick, stabilized babies. Now (2014), mothers and babies are kept together by having the RB&C Neonatal Intensive Care Unit just steps away from the MacDonald Women's Hospital's Maternal Fetal Medicine Unit. Dr. Kennell would be happy about that.

Child Life Flourishes

Always protective of programs supporting the needs of children, Dr. Kennell related that, at one point, he had a great concern:

> There were two pediatricians who thought about, or planned to discontinue Child Life. Those were very stressful times . . . One of them called together all the heads of clinical divisions. He asked the head of Child Life to provide all sorts of information and present a lot of data. This put great pressure on her, but she did it very well . . . After she finished speaking, Dr. Klaus and I spoke and had slides. Then the group was asked their opinion about discontinuing Child Life. Dr. Herndon, the chief of orthopedics at that time . . . raised up and said, "Are you suggesting that we get rid of the Child Life program? I wouldn't work a day in a hospital that didn't have a program like this. I insist that

every patient of mine have a child life worker!" He went on and on. The meeting closed soon after that. The Child Life program continued and flourished.

Ongoing financial support from the Rainbow Foundation, the group that started the Rainbow Hospital on Green Road, has secured patient- and family-centered Child Life as an integral part of Rainbow Babies and Children's Hospital. Dr. Kennell was always greatly supportive of the women of the Rainbow Board and has pointed out:

> That they've helped tremendously with the finances of Rainbow Babies and Children's Hospital. At first it was focused on the Child Life programs, but then it was gradually expanded as they wisely invested their money to help with many functions in the hospital.

Note: John Kennell quotations were taken from unpublished interviews conducted by Mary Hellerstein, MD on March 21 and August 23, 2007.

Chapter 9
BONDING: THE ATTACHMENT OF MOTHERS TO THEIR INFANTS

The Collaboration Begins

During his 1966 sabbatical in England, Dr. Kennell heard that Dr. Marshall Klaus was doing a study allowing mothers into the nursery with their infants and contacted him. Dr. Kennell had first met Marshall Klaus as a resident at Babies and Children's in 1952. Later, in the mid-1960s, Dr. Klaus became Director of the Clinical Research Center for Premature Infants at Stanford. While working on surfactant, along with other projects, he had begun to observe—and then turn his attention to—the mothers of the babies. He and his coworkers also did an interesting study that showed there were fewer pathogenic organisms in the nursery when mothers were present (Barnett, Leiderman, Grobstein, & Klaus, 1970) Dr. Klaus told an interviewer:

> When I came to Cleveland we just teamed up, John and I, because we were absolutely ready. He had looked at one aspect of sneaking them (mothers) in and saw a very different outcome . . . He's very gentle. You know John (Klaus, 2000).

When Dr. Kennell returned from sabbatical in 1967, Dr. Klaus had been hired to run the premature and newborn nursery. Dr. Kennell was responsible for the pediatric clinic and some private patients. Both men did research and soon began working together to study the benefits of allowing mothers to spend time with their infants in the premature nursery. Dr. Kennell thought contact should begin within the first week. This was based on his previous observations of mothers watching their infants through the window and later coming to visit their infants in an isolette.

In unpublished studies, they filmed mothers feeding their infants. Mothers who were allowed to touch their babies earlier were more regular about their visits than those who did not touch their baby for weeks or months. One early study (1970) was designed to photographically document normal maternal-infant behavior for both premature and full-term infants. The full-term infants were filmed for 10 min at the first meeting with the mother (an average of 5.3 hours). Eye-to-eye contact and palm contact developed rapidly within that time. For healthy premature infants, there was a similar sequence, but it occurred far more slowly. Even after three visits (the third averaging 5.1 days after delivery), mothers did not spend nearly as much time watching their babies and touching them as did the mothers of the full-term babies at their first meeting. The investigators suggested that the early postnatal period might be "especially sensitive for the development of close affectional ties in the human mother"(Klaus, Kennell, Plumb, & Zuehlke, 1970).

Multiyear Studies of Full-Term Babies

In the late 1960s, many of Dr. Kennell's studies were done in collaboration with medical students, who were enthusiastic about these opportunities. These studies were done during the summers when students had breaks. Follow-up studies could be done the following summer. Some of the students were distressed about their observations at McDonald House, the maternity hospital. They noted that mothers were not given the same care and attention on the staff service as on the private service. For example, there was less lighting on the staff unit. The students wanted this difference brought to the attention of the newspapers, radio stations, and TV stations of Cleveland.

Dr. Kennell told the students that first they had to do a study to document the need for changes. Still, the medical students had problems with this concept; they wanted all the patients to have the same care. Dr. Kennell gradually convinced them of the value of doing a randomized, controlled study. At this time, most mothers were given "twilight sleep" during the last stages of labor. This was a mixture of morphine and scopolamine, and was very powerful. Mothers had no memory of what went on. Many said and did things that would be embarrassing, had they known about them, such as swearing or taking off clothing. Due to the effects of these drugs, mothers were not able to care for their infants immediately after delivery, and infants often had problems breathing. Both mothers and infants required separate recovery areas with close attention for 12 to 18 hours.

The object of the initial study was to compare this traditional birth routine with mothers and babies who had early contact. Randomization was achieved by having all the full-term infants given one procedure for one month, followed by the alternate procedure the following month. At first, the researchers watched through an observation room window as infants received eye drops and vitamin K injections. The average time before the mother and infant could be brought together was 8 to 12 hours. Dr. Kennell and the medical students worked hard to reduce this time period. They had to overcome the objections of nurses and pediatric residents, who opposed changing the rules. Finally, they came to an agreement for this study; a nurse would bring the mother and father to the room with the study infant within the first 3 hours after delivery. The nude baby would be under an overhead heat panel to keep warm. Parents were there for 45 minutes and the nurse would enter every 15 minutes to check on how they were doing together. The slightest sound or evidence of a possible problem would cause the nurse to check again.

The usual procedure at that time was for the infants to be brought to the mothers for breastfeeding or bottle-feeding every 4 hours for 20 or 30 minutes. As Dr. Kennell noted:

This was not an ideal schedule for facilitating breastfeeding. A lot of mothers who were breastfeeding really didn't get a decent chance to succeed." In addition to these short visits, the early contact group had 5 hours of daily contact with the baby in the mother's room during her hospitalization. Some mothers stayed 3 days and some 4 days. These extra 5 hours per day of "rooming in" proved important.

A follow-up with mothers and their infants one month later included the usual questions about normal newborns, and also, questions related to the relationship of the mother with her baby. The results revealed that mothers with increased early contact were less likely to let their baby cry or leave the baby with someone else, and more likely to make eye-to-eye contact, soothe, and fondle the baby (Klaus et al, 1972). There were similar differences in the relationship of the mother with her baby when the infants were 1 year old (Kennell et al., 1974). It had taken a "heroic effort" to find all the families at one year. After that, the investigators decided that sending students into areas like Hough so soon after the riots was not really wise. Still, they carried out two later follow-up studies, when some of the infants were 2 and 5 years of age.

It was found that the increased contact group, by age 2, exhibited more complex communication patterns relative to controls (Ringler, Kennell, Jarvella, Navojosky, & Klaus, 1975). By age 5, the increased-contact infant group showed a close correlation between their language and that of the mothers speech at 2 years. This was not true for the control group (Ringler, Trause, Klaus, & Kennell, 1978).

Dr. Kennell once expressed that the first of these four studies (1972) was on the top of his list of important publications.The investigators had other concerns. Dr. Kennell explained:

We struggled over the words. We used "attachment" when we were planning all of it. But "attachment" is usually a term for the baby's relationship to the mother . . . Then we started saying that the process of the parent's attachment to the baby is "bonding," and the attachment of the infant to the mother is "attachment" because there is a lot of attachment literature.

While numbers were not large enough in those early studies to convince everyone about the need to provide mothers with early and extended infant contact, Dr. Kennell stated, "The study did show differences, so there was great excitement about the importance of early attachment that spread far and wide." These studies and similar ones from Stanford at the same time have been reviewed and updated in an article titled, "Parents in the Preterm Nursery and the Subsequent Evolution of Care"(Klaus & Kennell, 2004)

The Skeptics

Dr. Kennell and his colleagues hoped that early mother-infant contact would be introduced for all mothers, but some of the leading obstetricians were hardly convinced. Dr. Kennell remarked, "They said, 'you think there's an important difference, and we don't think it's that important'." There was a lot of skepticism, and many papers claimed that the findings were not convincing.

The indifference of their obstetric colleagues led Drs. Kennell and Klaus to design research that their colleagues might think of as more "important." The next chapter describes how their conclusions sent them in a new research direction, and led to new discoveries in the Latin American country of Guatemala.

Fortunately, publicity in newspapers and magazines about the impor-tance of early contact led parents to request increased contact with their infants. They began discussing this with obstetricians prior to the birth of their babies.

Gradually, the practice of allowing earlier infant contact spread throughout the United States. By the 1980s, most mothers expected that they would be allowed to room in with their new infants.

The caring and observational skills of Dr. Kennell, Dr. Klaus, and other staff empowered them to take chances, to challenge the conventional wisdom, and to advocate for what was best for mothers and babies. During the years, they were working in Guatemala, they put together a book on early contact, bereavement, and the time throughout pregnancy and the first weeks after birth. It also covered sick and challenged infants. The focus was on helping parents understand and care for themselves and their infants (Klaus & Kennell, 1976).

To maximize the accuracy, and to acknowledge the complex nature of these topics, the authors also included comments from 19 different investigators in related fields. This 1976 book was updated to more fully include the father in 1982 (Klaus & Kennell, 1982). However, in the first book, and one paper, the authors unwittingly set themselves up for great criticism regarding those first days after birth. As Dr. Klaus put it:

> In the book we suggest that this early period is unique for
> the mother and baby. That is she's open to change, and that
> it's a critical period. That word "critical" was a major error.
> It's a "sensitive" period. Critical means if it doesn't occur,
> all is lost. That created an immense amount of problems,
> which continues even to this day (2000) because nobody
> has read after that (second) book (Klaus, 2000)

It should also be pointed out that as early as the 1972 *New England Journal of Medicine* paper, Drs. Kennell, Klaus, and their colleagues had already dispensed with the term "critical period." The term was commonly used to denote the short period during which an infant is imprinted on, and thus attaches to a parent figure. Rather, in that paper, they sought a term for the widely investigated special period immediately after delivery in the adult animal that promotes characteristic mothering behavior. They proposed using the expression "maternal sensitive period." Multiple physiological interactions occur simultaneously between mother and infant under more natural conditions. It is a fail-safe reciprocal system that is overdetermined to insure the proximity of mother and infant (Kennell & Klaus, 1979).

Despite the growing appreciation for the supportive conditions that promote infant attachment and maternal bonding, the topic was once again challenged in the early 1980s. Seven different investigators then gave point-by-point responses to the criticisms. They detailed errors in the challenger's numbers, and in understanding the specific benefits for women with a lower level of social support. They also showed how some study designs were misinterpreted, and how important factors used in determining the significance of results were overlooked (Anisfield et al., 1983). Unfortunately, the harshness of the criticisms, the growing pressures of technology, and the natural variation among individual mothers and their circumstances discouraged investigators from pursuing additional bonding studies.

"Soft" science is a most difficult science.

Note: John Kennell quotations were taken from a series of unpublished interviews conducted by Mary Hellerstein, M. D. February 2 and April 20, 2007.

SECTION II

GUATEMALA AND THE DOULA STUDIES

Chapter 10

EXPERIENCE IN A
MAYAN INDIAN VILLAGE

First Impressions

It was becoming clear that the first hours after birth were very important for developing a healthy relationship between a mother and her baby. Even the layout of the new RB&C hospital, with rooming-in, reflected this new understanding, although, more and longer-term studies lay ahead. However, the obstetric colleagues of John Kennell and Marshall Klaus did not find enough significant data in the bonding studies to convince them to change their practices. Rather, they suggested that their pediatrician friends ought to do something useful. Knowing that science likes clear-cut measurements and outcomes, they were challenged to find an alterative approach for demonstrating the importance of the bonding of mothers to their babies.

Instead of abandoning their convictions that the experience of childbirth could be greatly enhanced, they finally listened to one of their Fellows, Roberto Sosa, from Guatemala. He had suggested, several times, that the researchers should come to his country, where they could study something less subjective, like breastfeeding. Widely acknowledged as beneficial, breastfeeding could be easily measured. Spurred by the recognition that they could not carry out controlled studies in the U.S. because there were so few breastfeeding mothers, they welcomed the opportunity to do studies in Guatemala, where most mothers were still breastfeeding, and where costs would be low. Therefore, Drs. Kennell and Klaus, and their wives, Peggy and Lois, all traveled to Guatemala in 1972 in order to understand what study opportunities might be available.

The prestigious Institute of Nutrition for Central America and Panama (INCAP) in Guatemala City, is well-known for its research, including development of a special high-protein food supplement for children from local ingredients, called Incaparina. Projects in Santa Maria Cauque, between 1959 and 1963, focused on improving medical care and hygiene; 1964 and 1972, on the impact of infection; and 1972 and 1976, on improving diet. Dr. Nevin Scrimshaw was the founding director, who had led the institute with great dedication between 1949 and 1961 and, notes Dr. Kennell, Dr. Scrimshaw had been just a couple of years ahead of him at the University of Rochester School of Medicine. He was recruited to MIT, but he would still come back at intervals. As a potential resource for their research, the investigators made a visit to INCAP, where few Americans now worked. It was clearly a place with a high-level of research, and a well-trained, experienced staff. Although, the two doctors had other requirements for their research, they were generously given an office at INCAP.

Dr. Roberto Sosa, the former Fellow in Pediatrics at RB&C, was incredibly helpful, and at the beginning, introduced Drs. Klaus and Kennell to practicing physicians in Guatemala. Dr. Kennell introduces Roberto's family:

Roberto Sosa's father was from the middle class. He was a wonderful man. Somehow through the system in Guatemala, he received his education, and became a very fine and reputable lawyer. He helped us with many issues along the way. His large beautiful home was in a well-to-do part of the city. It was within a compound surrounded by high walls and very sturdy gates. A man at the gate let people in and out. The Sosas were very generous when we were in Guatemala and we were fed well. There were times when our wives would go with us to Guatemala and stay with us at the Sosa's.

Roberto's mother was the sister of the first president of Guatemala, Juan Jose Arevalo, 1945 to 1951. I learned about him in various ways. He was a highly honored historian and writer, so throughout many of the Central and South American countries, he was well-known and revered. As the first president, he developed a constitution and procedures that are very much like the laws of the United States, and he had a good relationship with the people in the United States. At the end of the term in office, the president was through. Guatemala did not have a communist party at the time he was president. But that changed as soon as he left office. As time went on, I think he was concerned, and so were his sister and her family, about some of the developments that came with the increasing presence of United States. There were many CIA people, often in civilian clothes. They would usually be wearing some emblems or signs, but would look like an average foreigner.

It became quite evident that internal political strife was a growing problem, but Dr. Kennell and his colleagues proceeded with their studies. Ultimately, the country became too dangerous for the research workers, and the studies, as described below, had to be ended.

The Village of Santa Marie Cauque

The Mayan Indian village of Santa Maria Cauque was not far from Guatemala City, and had been a part of comprehensive INCAP studies on nutrition and infection since the late 1950s. Juan Urrutia, a clinical pediatrician, and Leonardo Mata, a Harvard-trained Ph.D., were two of the senior faculty at INCAP, and focused their research there. Dr. Kennell describes the setting and life there:

It became apparent that these impoverished Indians had been treated cruelly from the beginning. The Spaniards took the flat lands and hills that you might imagine plowing, even though some were steep. They relegated the Indians to the tops of the mountains, where crops did not grow well. If there were any trees, they were scrubby. So the villagers in Santa Maria Cauque, and in many other villages, made do with this very poor land. With very rudimentary tools, they would plant the corn and keep the weeds down.

There was always an open fire going inside the thin-walled, adobe huts with a hole in the ceiling. It was very smoky inside . . . The Mayan Indians didn't use pots and pans, but had a flat dish made of clay that they put over the fire. The women sat by the fire and tended the tortillas, flipping them with their hands. Their hands were thick skinned, and I'm sure there was a lot of burning along the way. The wealthier Indians might have a few chickens that would give them some protein in their diet, but there weren't big flocks of chickens.

Cultivating good health in this environment was as difficult as cultivating the land. Children were not abandoned, and seldom experienced corporal punishment, but they were subject to rounds of malnutrition, precipitated by infection (INFDC, 1995). Dr. Kennell related that in the dirt floors of the homes, as well as in the soil outside, the INCAP researchers had found every parasite known to man, and that good-sized families might be living in one small home.

It became apparent that while the huts appeared to look the same, and the adults and children looked the same, there were big differences when you looked closely. Dr. Urruita told me about two families . . . In general, they were both terribly poor. However, in one place things were untidy. The other place would be like a Shaker Heights residence, even with its poor dirt soil. In the first home . . . the children were forever getting sick and having complications. In the place I'm comparing to Shaker Heights, the people were good about getting whatever was available for the children, in terms of any checkups or immunizations. They followed through with medication when the children were sick. The difference between the medical status of the two families was astounding: one family was very healthy and the other had all sorts of difficulties.

Just as the landscape, living conditions and lack of resources were a challenge for the Indian villagers, research here faced its own challenges. Dr. Kennell could see that conducting clinical studies was going to be more difficult than he had anticipated. A summary of an INCAP intervention study in Santa Maria Cauque gives a glimpse of working in a village. Since the Indians' diet had already been carefully analyzed and found to lack certain nutrients, the study design was to fortify the diet of half the participants. In order to establish a relationship with all the people, the INCAP investigators first took turns going throughout the village, inquiring how each family was getting along. The two principle researchers then brought most of the Indians together and said,

> [W]e've found that your diet could be better. We would like to have your approval to grind your corn as you have done for a long time and we will put some additional food into it. For a whole year, we will return the ground corn the next day so you can make your tortillas.

Dr. Kennell elaborates on the course of the INCAP study:

> The two investigators would go house to house every day and ask, "How are you doing? How is the corn coming? How are you doing with the picking?" They asked about other problems they had heard about the day before. They had to

be kind and thoughtful because if something went wrong, the study would get the blame. The study proposal led to tremendous turmoil. Some people never participated, and others participated on and off . . . Some of the participants would get upset if there was some illness or problem or sign from the stars that would make them think they shouldn't participate ... Keeping in touch with the study families as well as with the ones that didn't participate (controls) required a lot of work.

Although, the 4-year INCAP study didn't show gains in nutritional measurements, such as the 6-month birthweight or growth rate, there were fewer days of infant illness, and less mortality in the group accepting the maximum 8% fortification (INFDC, 1995).

Another example of unexpected factors influencing a study was noted at a Symposium in London. The naturalistic behavior of mothers immediately after hospital delivery could not be studied in the same way that had been done in Cleveland. Observers and cameras inhibited the Indian mothers. Belief in the evil eye also had a negative effect (Klaus, Trause, & Kennell, 1975).

Observing Local Birthing Practices

At that time in Santa Maria Cauque, most births occurred 10 to 20 minutes after spontaneous membrane rupture, with most women on their knees during the birth. No special drugs, procedures, or hygiene precautions were used (except for sterilizing the umbilical cord). Despite early exposure to infectious agents, newborns were almost never symptomatic. Mothers would breastfed their babies up to 2 years or longer, and often had 10 children. There was no bottle-feeding, even though 33% of the families owned cattle (in 1971). Within 3 days, a mother would return to work, and carry her baby in contact with her body. Weaning food was introduced at 3 to 5 months, so this became one route for new infection.

Dr. Kennell describes a typical birth:

> The people were hard working, but they did have a celebration, Saints Day, which occurred almost once a month. The people taking care of a teenage mother figured out the date of conception by figuring out the feast that preceded onset of pregnancy. The way they did it was really quite accurate. A pregnant teenager would continue working in the field, as was done all day, every day in the hot sun. She would be cultivating around the corn and any other crops they had. When she had the onset of labor pains, the wise women who were always around, would say, "Just keep on working." When the pains became more severe, they would go to the home and meet the native midwife. Usually the mother's mother, and mother's mother-in-law were present, even if they did not get along perfectly. The ones we observed did get along well. In this little home, the mother would walk and walk. When the final urge came she delivered her baby... I was never allowed in until well after the "clean up."

> After delivery, a woman would instantly put a knitted hat on the baby. This was crucial because they had beliefs that the "evil spirit" could harm the newborn infant. Caps for newborn infants are a worldwide phenomenon, with variations. The belief was that if they got the hat on the baby early, the effects from the "evil spirit" would be interrupted ... After delivery, the cap stayed on all the time. The mother quickly received wraps to keep the baby warm. The mother and mother-in-law would be there and would be attentive to make sure the mother successfully breastfed. This was crucial because the only way the baby could be fed would be by the mother. The new mother would stay with her mother or mother-in-law for at least the first year. She would get wonderful teachings.

An unmarried sister, or an experienced woman, might also help the mother and guide her when problems developed.

Dr. Kennell observed that the women knit beautifully colorful materials. Since breastfeeding was so prevalent in their culture, most women wore a blouse called a guipil. It had a well-designed slit that would allow women who were breastfeeding to imperceptibly shift from one breast to the other.

While giving the George Armstrong Award Lecture in 1980, Dr. Kennell stated his appreciation for these native traditions:

> There has been a remarkably low incidence of breech deliveries, 0.7% in contrast to 2% or more quoted in most textbooks. Does this give us ideas about what we should study in birth centers? There is no doubt that modern obstetrics has made remarkable advances, and we do not want to lose the gains that have been made, but it is interesting to note that no preeclampsia or eclampsia were observed in any patient in Santa Maria Cauque during the 15 years of study. No cases of puerperal fever, and no deaths of the mother during childbirth or puerperium occurred. Who shows the way and who follows? (Kennell, 1980)

The Cleveland Team

As Drs. Kennell and Klaus began their studies in Guatemala in 1973, they assembled a team to assist them. In addition to the Cleveland group, they were fortunate to acquire three marvelous, skilled field workers who had been working for Dr. Berry Brazelton. This outstanding pediatrician had studied the impact of poor nutrition on infant behavior, and had recently left the country. He has written a tribute letter near the end of this book. In the beginning, the field workers didn't carry out assignments as planned, and it really upset the investigators. However, as Dr. Kennell relates,

You didn't realize it, but all of a sudden you realized they were stroking your shoulder and calming you down, and it really did work well, and you knew they knew what they were doing. They were awfully good.

Dr. Kennell continues with a description of the Cleveland group:

It was a break from college so my daughter, Susan, was there for 5 to 6 weeks, with several medical students that we had recruited and trained. There were two people that were not medically trained, and students who just had completed the first two years of medical school at Case Western Reserve University, so they had quite a bit of experience with mothers and babies. There's a lot of sophistication picked up in the first two years, even though students aren't working on the hospital divisions.

One bright woman had a mind of her own. She had done a lot of volunteer work in Central America, and was determined to go back to the Central American village she had worked at the summer before. With great trepidation, I let her take a bus back to that community. At that time, there were reports of political strife, and people being shot as they traveled across certain areas. I worried, but she returned safely. Interestingly, she had gone back to the village square where she had spent the previous summer giving immunizations. People there would come and say, "Oh, it's so good you are still here," even though she had been away a year.

One of the medical students was male and a bit older than the others. He originally worked for General Motors before he came to medical school, and General Motors was paying his way through medical school. He was marvelous with machines. He came along to be a driver and to contribute to our work after we started the study. He was a big help to me.

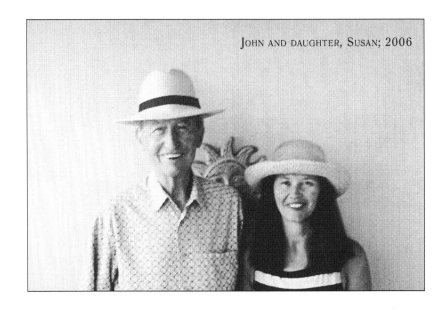

JOHN AND DAUGHTER, SUSAN; 2006

While nutrition was not the subject of their research, it did provide some stressful moments for the investigative team. Dr. Kennell stated:

> Marshall and I had thought about the dilemma of this group from Cleveland, one of whom came from California. They would be eating and living in Guatemala, and that could be risky. We worked out a plan; we would get meat and bread, and a few other items, and would prepare sandwiches for the students to take during the day. This way, they would eat safe food. However, one student was so independent that it was like being the parent of a rebellious teenager. She would say to the others, "You don't want to eat that stuff. Look, they have terrific food at the Central Market. Let's go and have a choice of all sorts of delicacies." At the end of the day they would come back, and we would all eat dinner together.

They would rave about their food and make disparaging comments about our white bread and dry meat. "It wasn't tasty." We also tried to advise everyone to be careful about what they drank. Then, after a few days, suddenly a few people were so sick with gastroenteritis that they couldn't go to work for a day or two. Everybody had assignments for the research study, and we didn't have backup people prepared to step in. So that was difficult. Some were very sick, including my daughter. I did not know at that time that she had Crohn's disease, and she was sick longer than the others. When they were well enough to come to the table a day or two later we talked about germs. It seems that what they were taught in the first two years of medical school hadn't registered. Still there were several who were far enough along in their training (we thought) to appreciate our precautions. Yet, every few days the same symptoms would keep one or more from the research work. It is important to report that the students worked diligently and offered valuable suggestions and observations. Fortunately, nobody acquired any persistent problems, except Susan.

Dr. Kennell describes a trip to Santa Maria Cauque when Susan accompanied the other students:

One of the INCAP doctors was helpful, but skeptical that Susan could do much, speaking only English. She kept saying, "I would love to do things with the children." Finally, he took her to a group of children in the village. He stayed around a while because he thought she was going to have a terrible time. But Susan had had experience with her little brother, and had a done a lot of babysitting. Almost instantly the kids gathered with her and played all sorts of games. When he came back he was astounded; he really thought she was something. She was planning to go into special education and work with children who had conditions, like Down syndrome.

In a letter home, Susan expressed how she had fallen in love with Santa Maria Cauque, and was thrilled to have the opportunity to be with her Dad in Guatemala. She wrote how the people were gracious, helpful, and bright, and how it would be difficult to leave.

The Rural Breastfeeding Study

In Santa Maria Cauque, the team participated in their first study on the relationship of breastfeeding and illness. It began in 1973 and was carried out as follows:

> As soon as the mother-to-be went home to give birth, the word went out, and our hired trained midwives would go to the home. They never entered the home, but stayed outside, and listened to the mother's screams. This way they could time what happened. They would remain there and talk to the native midwife and then one of the mother figures and even the mother, although that would be unusual. We had to be very careful about not violating any of the rules earlier investigators had established. The Mayan Indian mothers were very friendly with us even though we couldn't communicate. They came to like the "gringos." We were called that because we looked different from the INCAP investigators.

Data from this village study, along with latter studies, revealed a lower rate of infectious illness (rate per 100 child-weeks) among infants of breast-feeding mothers in both the rural (11.4) and urban settings (9.7) relative to urban infants who were not breastfed (16.8; Urrutia, Sosa, Kennell, & Klaus, 1979).

Chapter 11
WORKING IN GUATEMALA CITY

As the investigators thought more and more about their research plans, they envisioned studying what would happen to different mothers and their babies randomly assigned to different treatments in a hospital. They wanted to focus on how the baby did on its first year. While INCAP was a fine resource, the two doctors needed to look elsewhere. Consequently, most of the investigations were carried out in Guatemala City. Dr. Kennell describes the setting and the politics:

> We rented a house on the top of a very high plateau. From the front you looked out over the whole of Guatemala City and could see for miles. Off to the left was the airport that was important in the history of Guatemala. In the 1950s, the U.S. was very anxious about communists. In 1952, the Guatemalan Party of Labor, a communist party, gained legal status. The President of the United States and Secretary of State were worried about communism. I think there was also pressure from the banana companies and other profitable ventures. So during the Eisenhower presidency, the Americans invaded Guatemala, forcing President Jacobo Arbenz Guzman (1951 to 1954) to resign. There were a lot of people still around who could tell you about seeing

the U.S. planes come. They took over the airport and the roads. Carlos Castillo Armas (1954 to 1957), who became the president, was an Army man and he put the army first. He did unbelievably little for the poor Indians.

The political legacy of the country and the political climate at the time left an imprint on the minds of the investigators. Dr. Kennell explained:

Within a week of arriving in Guatemala with our medical students, we had a frightening experience. We were shown the day's paper. On the front page was a big picture of an 8-year old child with multiple wounds. He was on a stretcher and was being treated at one of the hospitals. The article said that a group of boys had found all sorts of guns and bullets and grenades right outside the estate where we were staying. These boys had apparently found the weapons, and not knowing anything about them fooled with them and had been injured.

There was a long, steep, winding road to get to our house on top of the hill and a gate at the entrance. We didn't want anyone to know Americans were there. An awful lot of people don't read, but I'm sure word of mouth and pictures put the idea across. All this was very worrisome to Marshall, Roberto, the students, and me. Was this a sign that people were getting ready to do something harmful to us? We were responsible for all of these students, in addition to the helper in the house.

We prevailed upon Roberto to call and ask his father, a highly regarded, honest lawyer to find out about this incident. His father said, "Yes, I'll find out and get back to you." A half hour later his father called back and said, "don't worry, they weren't after you." That was reassuring, but we weren't completely settled. The police by that time had taken away all the weapons. We came to realize that there were many places along the highway where people would be stopped and their car would be searched. The group carrying the weapons had probably been moving this equipment, and when they encountered a checkpoint, they quickly deposited the weapons and disappeared. We were told all the boys recovered. They had multiple bullet wounds.

During all of this we learned that one of the student's fathers was the head of a big pharmaceutical company. We were terrified that word would get out and someone might want to take the student hostage. Fortunately that did not happen, but we were all very careful about not talking to others.

Study Hospitals

The team sought out two hospitals in Guatemala City, Roosevelt Hospital, and the Social Security Hospital, for their randomized trials. For a year after delivery, they planned to study mothers and babies who had either early contact or the standard delivery-with-separation protocol. They would focus on measures of behavior, breastfeeding, and infection. These hospitals had, as Dr. Kennell describes enormously large delivery rates. "The babies we saw were healthy newborns. There were other clinics where sick babies were seen."

> People in Guatemala who had a job and an employer and were receiving pay on a regular basis for a year were eligible for what they called Medicare. That entitled them to deliver babies at the Social Security Hospital. When we first went to Guatemala it was the more friendly hospital of the two and all the women who went there were better off: better

clothing and better nourished. The very poor people went to Roosevelt Hospital. Some came from Indian villages, but a great many had left their Indian villages because there was not enough food.

We had an arrangement with the Roosevelt Hospital where we did most of our research. The hospital was built under the impetus of President Franklin Roosevelt just as the United States was entering WWII. As a college and medical student, I read that experts anticipated that the war would occur basically from the East. Therefore, ships would need to get through the Panama Canal. It would be disastrous for the United States if a Pacific fleet was needed and they couldn't get through the canal. It was anticipated that there would be a large number of soldiers stationed there, and there would need to be facilities for wounded people, yet not where planes would be bombing all the time. They picked Guatemala City although it was a quarter mile away, so the United States built a quarter mile of the Continental Highway. At that time the area was probably tremendously appealing because of its natural beauty, but the beauty was overwhelmed by development by the time I went there in 1972. The hospital was built to accommodate soldiers, but after the war it became an obstetric building. It was overcrowded, but had been well built. The hospital was given to the Guatemalan government after the war, but the government was poor. Early after the war I think there was much more interest in the Indians because they had been soldiers in the war and in Central America. Our government gave quite a bit of money to Guatemala, but I don't think it benefitted Indians.

The obstetricians at the Roosevelt hospital were remarkably sensitive and skilled (I don't know about all their training). They were very thoughtful of the poor people. They seemed to have the knowledge and ability to do things that we were doing in the United States, but without our technology. In the labor and delivery area there were often two types of nurses, one head nurse who had to be very knowledgeable, and one or two other nurses. I'm sure all the nurses were doing their activities faster than anybody in the U.S. can imagine.

There were a large number of new mothers every day, maybe 30 to 50. This number of deliveries was unbelievable for the size of the staff. The obstetric unit was so busy that three mothers might be delivering at the same time. The one man responsible for cleaning rooms following each delivery swished his mop back and forth so fast that it was a blur. The hospital's procedures had been set up by nurses and doctors from the United States in the 50s, and had not changed since then. Everything was very limited, and often there was just one sheet for a woman. They did not have epidural analgesia, but this was also not generally available in the U.S. at that time. This was an environment where poor people without prenatal care were coming so there was a very high incidence of toxemia. Several patients came in having seizures. Despite using procedures that were standard in Cleveland many of the mothers were too ill to survive.

Study Procedures

Recruiting for a study was carried out in many stages. Dr. Kennell begins with the community of La Florida:

While Guatemala City had some streets and beautiful buildings there were also a tremendous number of huts people put up on the edge of the city, many on the sloping sides of hills. Areas that had been occupied for quite a while had become organized, and there were streets and buildings. We had been told to pick mothers from La Florida, which was out farther. The population must have been large. The people that lived in the houses had stores and a very tiny central community. We had to talk with the mothers, so Marshall and I took some Spanish lessons. I did the best I could do with what I had been taught. We would ask if they had come from La Florida, and a few details about the pregnancy and fetus. We only selected mothers having their first baby and the pregnancy had to be progressing normally. The mothers were often quiet. Once I turned around after I had just been asking these questions. All the women were laughing behind their hands at my Spanish attempt to ask if they were from La Florida. I was aware that my Spanish was not very good. It was an embarrassing experience. Later when we were not in Guatemala our researchers did the questioning and recruiting.

At Roosevelt Hospital most of the mothers would have come to the hospital door; it was not an elegant door—just a back door. Someone would say there is a mother and they would figure out she was having a baby. They would admit her, but keep the family out. Excluding family members was totally different than what went on in the Indian villages. The mother was taken into a building she had never been in, taken to a floor she had never been on, and finally left in a tiny room by herself. There she would labor and deliver her baby. The mothers were terrified, particularly when they went into active labor. They were crying (in Spanish), "Help me, save me, operate, do a cesarean." We were at the hospital all the time looking for patients like that who were about to deliver. They don't all go at the same speed. We would be alert to a mother who had just come in since she might be the next one who would deliver. So we kept circulating around. The women were really alone, and when they had pains they were screaming and frantic. It was awful. Then the women who had just delivered would be waiting to be put into a bed. They might have to wait a long time since it depended on other mothers being discharged.

Our researchers were told not to spend time in a delivery room. One of them would get permission from the mother to just explain our study, saying she might have time with her baby right after delivery, or she might get her baby later. Then another researcher would attend the delivery. We didn't sign them up until we had watched the first few minutes and saw that the baby and the mother were doing well. It was very important to find a time when she was peaceful enough to ask if she would participate in the study. The mothers were wonderful about participating and most of them agreed. That's different than going to the village and asking if we could put something in their food. In general, the women were very short and thin, with zero obesity. The babies were small and thin, and 4.5 lbs. was the average weight for a full-term baby. The baby's skin looked like the wrinkled skin of post-mature babies. You rarely see this now in the United States. It became thicker after a day or two, and then began to peel. The malnutrition that had been identified so clearly by INCAP was affecting these women and their babies.

Random assignments would tell whether the mother would have early contact with her baby or not. We planned to put a slip in the same type of envelope that had worked wonderfully in the U.S., one you couldn't see through. Fortunately we discovered early on that the sun in Cleveland was not like the bright sun in Guatemala. Someone found that if you looked up at the sky you could see through the brown envelope. From then on we put in black paper as a shield. For early contact the researchers would go down the hallway with the mother and into an empty room, and for controls (routine hospital procedure), they would be given assignments in which mothers wouldn't get together with their baby until several hours later. It was not ideal, but it was set up that way because of the study we had done on bonding in Cleveland. (At that time, the breastfeeding rate in the U.S. was very low. It was lowest in 1960, and the rate didn't increase much until later. So all the mothers that had been in that Cleveland study did not breastfeed and did not have early skin-to-skin contact.)

We brought a heat shield to put over the newborn, early contact babies in the hospital to keep the baby warm. While you may think of Guatemala as hot, it was cold at night.

When we shut the door to the laboring woman's room, we had no way to look in. We would come back 45 min to 1 hour later to see the mother with the baby (the experimental group). We weren't sure if the mother breastfed or not, but it was extremely probable that all mothers had breastfed their babies. Then the baby had to be moved to a different location to be checked in by the nurses. In general, babies on the division of healthy babies and mothers would be in the nursery and be examined. Any questions would be checked by one of us physicians. Both groups would be on a friendly ward, where the mothers could get up and walk around with their babies, talk with other mothers, and breastfeed their babies. All the mothers had to breastfeed. They would be there from 9 to 9:30 in the morning (after examination of all the babies in the nursery had been completed) until 5 or 6 p.m. The routine was quite progressive compared to the United States. While they had a small number of nurses, mothers with problems could get more attention. I thought they did that well.

On the Road: The Bus

Dr. Kennell reveals how every aspect of the study required special attention, including travel:

> From our visits to Guatemala, and our correspondence, we realized we needed a bus. It was crucial to get to a village to take a mother and baby home after they were discharged from the hospital; then we would know the name of that lane or path where the mother lived so we could keep track of the baby. If you went to some of these places as a gringo you would have a terrible time finding it.

> With the help of INCAP, we obtained a VW bus. They generously provided gas and oil and service. The roads were unbelievably severe. I don't think any U.S. car, other than a VW bus, would have lasted more than a few days. When we first went to Guatemala it was sunny and warm, but much of the year was rainy. When it was rainy and you went to a home, you encountered big potholes that were hard to recognize in the big puddles. The whole bus would almost

tip over, leaning hard to the right or to the left repeatedly. Fortunately our drivers were excellent.

Our team would take a scale to weigh the baby. They would spend time to get to know the people who were living nearby. Employers frequently moved the villagers and neighbors were likely to be able to inform our Guatemalan research workers where to find the baby and mother. It's a great thing about Guatemalan culture (something we've lost in our country); even though people were very busy in Indian villages, there was always a woman to take care of the babies and children.

Chapter 12
EXPANDING UNDERSTANDING: THE DOULA STUDY

Study Results

For research purposes, the mothers and babies were followed in their own community, and, as Dr. Kennell explains:

> We found early on that we had to be very attentive to
> how babies were doing in their homes. Our Guate-
> malan research workers were very helpful with this. For
> example, they had a mother whose baby was well below
> the birth weight. They talked with the mother and learned
> that she was terribly poor. She had no money or way of
> getting food, but was getting something about once a day
> for herself. Understandably, the baby was very thin. We
> thought this was an emergency, and the U.S. response
> in us was to immediately get some Similac or Enfamil for
> the baby. Then we quickly became realistic. How was
> this poor mother who couldn't get food for herself, going
> to get formula? We were very anxious about this (the
> case is written up). So we arranged for the diet of the
> mother to be greatly enhanced. We had to be cautious
> because she had gone so long without adequate food. It

went all right with her but there was still nothing for that poor baby for the first three or four days. Finally, the mother had more milk. Once the mother had adequate milk and food for herself, she produced adequate breast-feeding milk for her infant. That was one of the babies we kept following. As I recall the baby did well during the study year.

Dr. Kennell and his coworkers were encouraged as they continued their studies. They "did the research in several different ways and there were benefits from the mother having the baby early." Research published from Roosevelt Hospital demonstrated effects of the early mother-infant contact on behavior after birth. The mothers who had skin-to-skin contact with their babies for 45 mins immediately after birth (experimental group) were significantly more affectionate at 36 hours than mothers who first received their wrapped babies at 12 hrs. (control group). This included looking at, talking to, fondling, kissing and smiling at the baby (Hales, Lozoff, Sosa, & Kennell, 1977).

Other studies examined breastfeeding and infections in mothers at 1, 3, 6, 9, and 12 months at both the Roosevelt and the Social Security Hospitals. Compared with controls, a higher percentage of mothers in the early contact group were breastfeeding at every time point and experienced a significantly longer duration of breastfeeding. Their babies also had fewer infections. Finally, it was especially pleasing for the early-contact mothers to see their babies looking at them, since the silver nitrate eye drops (for preventing infection) had been delayed until 45 minutes after birth (Sosa, Kennell, Klaus, & Urrutia, 1976).

Dr. Klaus has pointed out that a number of the Guatemalan studies were published in three different CIBA Symposia, where they were not as easily available as they would have been in journals. He felt this was a mistake because skeptics were not able to examine details of the studies. In six of nine studies from seven countries between 1976 and 1981, there was significantly more breastfeeding at 2 or 3 months postpartum if mothers had early suckling and breastfeeding during the first hour of life (Sosa, Kennell, Klaus, & Urrutia, 1976). These studies may not have specifically proven that longer breastfeeding indicates better mother-to-infant bonding, but they gave support to the Baby-Friendly Hospital Initiative (BFHI) that is an existing global program of the World Health Organization and the United Nations Children's Fund. In this program, breastfeeding is the focus of practices to improve infant health. Countries with the program, such as Thailand and Costa Rica, have seen a dramatic decrease in the abandonment of babies in maternity hospitals. Dr. Klaus also has spoken of a seldom-mentioned benefit of breastfeeding; it increases the baby's stooling that, in turn, promotes bilirubin excretion.

The Presence of Other Women during Delivery: Prelude to the Doula Study

Here is a bit of background for the amazing incident that will be described shortly. Dr. Kennell explains:

> Anthropologists have confirmed the success of having someone present with the mother during labor and delivery. We reviewed 128 nonindustralized cultures where there was data (Murdock and White, 1969). It was a marvelous source of information current through the 1960s to 1970s. I assume it is still true of the majority of deliveries throughout the developing world. There were details from these 128 cultures that revealed whether the mother labored alone or with someone. All but one of these cultures had someone present with the mother. That included a variety of people with a variety of training and experience. The team needed a term to apply to the person helping a mother during labor and during that time we were reading a book by Dana Raphael about breastfeeding.

She referred to a person she called a doula who helped mothers after the baby was born and recommended that doulas should be developed to help support and promote breastfeeding (Raphael, 1973).

Doula is a modern Greek word. In Greece, wealthier families would have a slave who would be responsible for taking care of the baby right after birth and probably a long time after that. As time passed, the idea of having someone with the mother continued. The person changed from being a slave to being a servant, but the same word doula was continued. This concept continued into the 18th to 20th century. It usually meant a woman present and often several women. We chose the word even though we didn't like the slave connotation. We've also emphasized the time period throughout labor and delivery and shortly afterwards, including time for skin-to-skin contact with the mother and breastfeeding.

Dr. Kennell himself had an early introduction to childbirth, and it made him think about whether support from another woman during labor might help the women in urban Guatemala too.

I spent my first summers with my wonderful grandmother on her farm. I had the experience on a few occasions of her telling me in the morning that she had been out during the night with other women. Once they had assisted at a birth when my playmate Tim's new brother was born. My grandmother was not trained, but she had attended many births. People knew that, and she would be contacted. I think several people were usually present. I was only a little boy. It was a big deal to me to think about somebody being present at the delivery of a baby.

Dr. Klaus' wife, Phyllis, also has spoken on the topic:

> The traditional midwife is a daya in Egypt ... The whole concept is that the midwife herself often wants the support of another woman. The woman would be the mother or mother-in-law or sisters. It would often be somebody who had much experience in childbirth. I interviewed a group of 9 daya in Egypt. These were wonderful women who maybe delivered 7 or 8 babies a night. They are so busy, but they would show how the women would surround the mother and sing with her, and chat with her, and help her into different positions. She would never be left alone. She would be totally supported and they absolutely recognized the importance of this. But, of course, this is true in many countries. We isolated women, which was a mistake (Klaus, 2000).

An Unexpected Result

Who can say why the unplanned happens at a perfectly timed moment, so that an idea grows beyond the mere anecdotal footnote? Once again, a carefully designed protocol was disregarded, to the dismay of the researchers. The medical students had been told that they had to do things according to hospital rules and to not interfere. This meant that the researchers must not be involved with any mother until after delivery, when permission was obtained for her to be in the study, that even then, they should not go into the room or talk with the mother.

One of the students, Karen Wendy Freed, did not follow protocol. Once a mother was admitted into the bonding study, she felt she shouldn't leave the mother alone. She would go in and talk with them, and would stay there. She spoke Spanish fluently. These particular mothers all received their babies right after birth.

When Wendy discussed the first 10 babies after joining the study, she acknowledged to Dr. Klaus that the mothers were very calm and peaceful. It seemed as though a number of things were better for these mothers. The 10 babies involved were not randomized or included in the data.

As Dr. Kennell reports:

> The positive outcome of the babies was striking, but we didn't know if it was a fluke. Very often, when you see something different that you think is going to be marvelous, there is a simple explanation that does not give you valuable new information. Therefore, we proceeded to design a new study for confirmation. For this study, Dr. Klaus and I had Dr. Roberto Sosa as our collaborator. He soon became our most valued collaborator in Guatemala. He not only had a private pediatric practice, but he also looked after the babies at the Roosevelt Hospital, as well as at the Social Security Hospital. He would check all the babies that had been enrolled in the study the day before and do the discharge exam. He also helped with several other studies. I don't think anybody else could have done all that he did. We were very fortunate.

Doula Studies: An Old Idea Takes Birth

Dr. Kennell continues:

> We planned a new randomized trial very carefully. It included 20 mothers in each group. In the study, one of our research women would became the doula and would open the envelope to find out the random assignment. We did not give this information to other people. The doula would know, but she would tell no one. Our

research doulas were absolutely marvelous: bright, enthusiastic, creative, and dependable. We had a good system, and our three research workers were wonderful in their understanding and reliability. They had had no experience with obstetrics or pregnancy, but they learned quickly. They were instructed to sit in the mother's room, and be attentive and friendly. Each month, the doulas and Dr. Sosa would collect the information about the mothers and babies, and we would get together to go over the data. We couldn't share the accumulating information with others, as that would spoil the study. The results showed remarkable differences between the mothers who labored alone and mothers who had a doula.

Including only the 40 mothers and neonates with normal, uncomplicated labor and delivery, the study showed that the doula-supported mothers had labored half as long as the control mothers (9 vs. 19 hours). Following delivery, mothers in both groups had been given their babies for the first 45 minutes. The ones who had a doula slept significantly less and spent a significantly greater percentage of the time they were awake in stroking, smiling, and talking with their babies. An assessment of all recruited mothers revealed fewer problems overall for the doula supported mothers (Sosa, Kennell, Klaus, Robertson, & Urrutia, 1980).

Dr. Kennell noted that when he and his colleagues discussed these differences, they immediately felt they had to do a larger study to be certain of their findings. It was also carried out at the Social Security Hospital. They anticipated that implementing such a study would give clearer results with more significant differences due to a larger sample. Roberto Sosa, who already had been so crucial, made sure the data collection went along and was completed. The earlier results were confirmed. As before, the mothers with doulas labored less than half as long as did mothers who had no support during labor (7.7 vs. 15.5 hours). The report in 1986 detailed the significant decreases in both the number of cesareans (6.5% vs. 17.3%) and the use of oxytocin (2.4% vs. 13.3%). The percent of supported mothers who had complications was half that of mothers without a doula and many fewer babies had difficulties (Klaus, Kennell, Robertson, & Sosa, 1986).

"Unfortunately," Dr. Kennell related, "as we told obstetricians in the United States about our results, we realized that we were not going to impress them, if we did not do our research in the United States. Leaders in obstetrics whom we talked to would say, 'Those are Guatemalans in Guatemala, and it doesn't relate to the United States. We aren't going to change what we do.'"

Chapter 13
A DIFFICULT ENVIRONMENT

Earthquake

E arthquakes are an intimate part of the story of Guatemala. Dr. Kennell explains:

> The whole country is built on volcanoes and they are still active. The area where we worked was very volcanic. Whenever we were there, there was at least one active volcano. When it became active in the dark you would see the flames coming from the volcano. The very first time we went to Guatemala in 1972, a volcano erupted, and it was severe enough that big black clouds covered the sky. We had gone to a beach house that belonged to Roberta Sosa's family. They had warned us to be very careful and stay under the trees because "the sun is so bright that you will get burned." So we were staying under the trees while we were reading our books. We noted that other people were flicking things off their pages. We didn't think much about it until we began feeling cold, even though we were supposed to be so hot! A cloud of volcanic ash had come overhead and began to block the sun. In a very short time, there was quite a thick layer of ash on everything including the car

we were driving. Guatemala had a very severe earthquake in 1976. I was not there and I have not seen the village of Santa Maria Cauque since that earthquake. I learned that largely due to the thin adobe clay walls, all the homes in the village of Santa Maria Cauque were totally destroyed, completely flattened. There was a very high mortality of children and parents. However, there were many babies in that village and they all survived. This was of interest to me because of all the discussions in the United States about whether babies should sleep with their parents. Even though many mothers died from the falling adobe, the babies were protected.

Dr. Kennell continues with the aftermath of the earthquake:

During our work there we didn't have any communications with the Mayan chiefs in the village, but there was a large building that you could say was the "administrative headquarters" of Santa Maria Cauque. There were often two or three male Mayan Indians who would be sitting on the porch and did not appear to be doing anything. However, after the earthquake these men turned into balls of fire. They went for 48 to 96 hours steady. They immediately grabbed several people and prepared signs saying, "Help! Help! Help! All our buildings are destroyed! Many children and adults dead! Please come with emergency assistance." And they sent people with signs out to the highways to stay there and see if they could get somebody to help assist. They organized service groups to go different places to see if they could rescue anybody. They also wanted to have a count of the people who died. They began digging graves right away.

Before the third day was over, the village was sort of back to normal. All of the dead were buried, everyone who was alive was back to working in the fields. Ironically, at the end of the day, the three men were back sitting on the porch. The Mayan Indians have a history of many earthquakes and many losses, so they are able to handle things in an impressive way. Then a great many people came from other places to help Santa Maria Cauque. A large group of Swiss built beautiful houses so that the village changed from adobe to very nice wooden Swiss-like structures. Other groups also built houses there. The Mayan Indians weren't thrilled with the Swiss: they were so religious, sober, and hard working. They liked the Americans better.

At the time of the earthquake, Dr. Kennell explains that in Guatemala City:

Dr. Sosa not only had a private practice, but also was taking care of our research throughout most of the year. There were the two hospitals and he would have to go to both places and check babies who were due to go home. He would also check how the research workers were doing there and what deliveries they had had. This was quite time consuming. The patients at the Social Security Hospital had better beds, better facilities, and more nurses. The building was very large and impressive. I don't know what it was originally. Before the earthquake they kept the babies in the nursery 12 hours at night, and while they had many nurses, they only brought the babies out three times a day for the mothers. The mothers with the Medicare program could get free milk. It seemed like such a great thing for Guatemalans, so most of the mothers were bottle-feeding. The food they laid out for the mother would be excellent by Mayan standards: a big portion of chicken, mashed potatoes, and other things. They planned very wisely. For women it was a good meal to have after having a baby.

The devastation in Guatemala City was quite severe and the Social Security Hospital was structurally, very damaged. Aftershocks, although, only lasting a few seconds, could go on for a long time, causing further damage. This meant there was no possibility of getting 50 or 100 babies out of the hospital and into the street; it was just impossible. So, similar to what was being done at Roosevelt Hospital, they closed the nursery and put the babies in bed with the mothers with all the beds touching one another. Dr. Kennell notes that:

> Everyone just had to climb over beds. By having the babies in bed with the mother, the incidence of infection, which was a very big problem in Guatemala, declined dramatically (Urrutia et al., 1979). We had been keeping track of the terribly high rate of very serious infections. I don't know how Roberto Sosa did all of the exams at that place. Ultimately, the babies and the mothers were moved to another place. It was an old rehabilitation hospital, and was not designed for mothers to labor and deliver, but people made do with that.

Dr. Kennell continues on to explain how Roberto Sosa's family had a difficult time during the earthquake.

> The family's response was characteristic of most people in Guatemala. They had a big place with large trees, a beautiful lawn, high walls, and a high fence. Roberto had three very impressive brothers who lived in their own homes. There were several people working at his place. Roberto's mother was a very able, wonderful woman, and she and some of the nieces and nephews were there. Roberto Sosa and his wife were living nearby. While the house was well built, the earthquake caused some damage, and there was fear that a later tremor might cause the place to collapse, so they moved outside onto the lawn. After the earthquake, Roberto Sosa had to get up extra early to go to both hospitals. Then

he would return to see how his family was doing. Every night and every morning he would say, "one or two of you have to go to the Red Cross to get emergency rations. The rest of you have to get some bedding or whatever we need and some of you have to get additional food for us." There were many people there so they required quite a lot of food and water. He would come back pretty tired at the end of a day, often in the evening, and nobody had done anything. The earthquake had immobilized them. It did that to a lot of people. Roberto's brother in law was a physician psychiatrist, and I think his wife was there. They just couldn't get moving; it's surprising that even a doctor couldn't get moving. So Roberto would have to go out and get in line. By the time he got to most places the food and drink was gone. He had a hard time with that.

Support after the earthquake came in many different forms.

Dr. Scrimshaw's daughter Susan was an anthropologist in Los Angeles. She was a very impressive, energetic young woman, and as a member of this family had spent a long time in Guatemala. She was very dedicated to INCAP. Although she had an important appointment and research in California, the minute she heard about the earthquake, she got on the phone to make arrangements to fly to Guatemala to help. She brought supplies and support and appropriate materials for typing and so forth. She quickly surveyed what was there and talked to people. She wrote four big grants within a very short time after she arrived, typing night and day. She flew to Washington to submit them just under the deadline. She understood what was going to be more important for everybody even though the immediate situation was more urgent.

Guerrillas

Guerrillas were problematic both in destabilizing Guatemala and in giving the investigators reason to be anxious for their safety. Dr. Kennell elaborates on the situation:

> When we got to Guatemala, we began to hear about guerillas, but people were being nice to us and we didn't hear too much about them. Once there, we began to hear that problems with the guerillas were increasing. A large portion of the Guatemalan army was Indian. They didn't have a voluntary system or a draft for the army. At a young age, maybe 17 or 18, they were forced to go into the army. They were treated very roughly, comparable to young people in some of the African armies. Also it wasn't long before many of the Indians were accused of being guerrillas. Some had to become guerrillas to survive, but it was not their initial intention. They had learned over centuries they had to cooperate.

> Many of the doctors we met didn't have much understanding about what was going on. It became clear that the army and/or guerillas did cruel things in Indian villages and this grew worse and worse. For example, they would fly over a village as if they were dropping water or fertilizer, but with their machine guns they would kill a large number of the Mayan Indians, women, children, and babies. Since there were a great many villages, it was hard to keep track of it all.

> Another tactic would lead to wiping out an entire village: several part Indian or Hispanic people would come to a village and say, "you have to help us; the armies are after us and they've killed our family and friends. You have to

help us; could you give us something?" The Indians would become suspicious, but then they would yield. They would be nice and give them a little food and water. Then all of a sudden there would be guerilla soldiers saying, "here you are helping the government soldiers, so we're going to punish you and kill everybody" or all the women or all the men or whatever. Many Indians were tricked that way.

The Guatemalan Situation Worsens

The political situation in Guatemala became progressively worse. Each time the Clevelanders would return to Guatemala, they learned from their field workers and the INCAP staff that the guerilla problem and the fighting was becoming more dangerous. Everything in the papers was about how terrible the guerillas were. The army was getting tougher and tougher on the guerillas. Similar battles were going on in Nicaragua too. In both countries, it was the poor people doing the fighting.

One serious incident took place at INCAP, where they routinely held grand rounds, which included visiting lecturers and interesting cases. One day, in 1980, in the middle of a meeting, half the audience got up and stood next to the walls around the room. Under their white coats they had guns. The leaders asked for the person in charge. Although no one answered, they figured it out. They kidnapped Dr. Carlos Tejada, the third director of INCAP (1975 to 1980), as well as INCAP's Administrator Richard Newman, who was a hematologist with whom Betsy Lozoff had done research. They made everybody stay there a long time while they took people away. Fortunately, no one from Cleveland was present. Dr. Kennell continues:

> The two men were in captivity for quite a long time. Perhaps the guerillas hoped that the fame of INCAP hostages would result in the world condemning the cruel Guatemalan army. After many days, negotiations began

for money for the release of these two. I don't know whether any money actually came forth. The men were told they would be freed, but they would have to leave Guatemala with all their family and possessions within 24 hours. These two men, whose lives had been totally involved with INCAP for years, had to move. There was a lot of publicity. During this time, several INCAP people disappeared and were killed. Some were found. Everybody could see that things were getting worse.

As Dr. Kennell reports, the research in Guatemala had to be closed in 1983::

Our field workers included a driver and two others who went along to take mothers home. In the city of Guatemala, they could rarely go more than two blocks without being stopped by some guerilla group. They would order the people out and up against the side of the VW bus, and would search them and shove them around a little bit. That and many other things made it clear to us that these three wonderful field workers could be injured or killed. We talked with them about it. Two had friends in the United States, so they went safely to the United States. The third one was married and she decided to stick it out. She did survive. We had to stop all research activities. Fortunately, we already had a lot of crucial data, but other projects were underway that we could never do.

Note: John Kennell quotations (chapters 10-13) were taken from unpublished interviews conducted by Mary Hellerstein, MD on 4/20/2007, 4/26/2007 and 5/3/2007 as well as a February 1995 interview by Susan McGrath for SRCD.

Chapter 14
RETURN TO THE UNITED STATES: DEVELOPMENT AND IMPLEMENTATION OF THE DOULA STUDIES

Background

In order to extend the doula research, it was important to do a project in a hospital in the United States that was similar to the study in Guatemala. Unfortunately, in U.S. hospitals at that time, the trend was to have the father of the baby present in the labor and delivery suite. This would produce a confounding variable. The irony here is that both Drs. Kennell and Klaus would have appreciated this trend in view of their passion to improve the care of the mother and her baby. Still, they needed to find a U.S. hospital with enough deliveries per year to make a doula study feasible, but one that did not permit the presence of family members during labor and delivery. That was not an easy task in the early 80s. They did locate a hospital in Tampa with enough deliveries, so they designed a pilot study to begin in 1983. However, just as the investigators were working out the details with obstetricians and nurses on the labor and delivery unit, the hospital changed its policy. Now family members were to be allowed in the labor and delivery unit at all times. So, between the time when they first started thinking about Tampa as a possible study site, until the time they received the grant money, hospital policy changed. The Tampa study never began.

Houston I

Therefore, Drs. Kennell and Klaus once again began the search for a hospital with limited visiting for family members. By 1982, Dr. Klaus had become Professor and Chairman of the Department of Pediatrics and Human Development at Michigan State University. Still, he would work with Dr. Kennell on studies. Fortunately, in Houston, they located Jefferson Davis Hospital, which had a very busy maternal care program. There, the Chief of Obstetrics, Clark Hinkley, allowed the team to carry out their doula study.

Susan McGrath, an associate investigator, joined the study in the summer of 1984, just as the team moved to Houston. Susan reports:

> It was a huge public hospital and I think they had about 13,000 deliveries per year ... an incredible number. At the time, our hospital had about 3,000. The hospital basically served a low-income, transient, Hispanic population, so most of the women who delivered at that hospital were either on public assistance, or had no medical insurance at all. Many of them were probably illegal ... although they were very careful not to reveal that to us ... I would guess that about half of them did not have English as their primary language.

For Susan, Houston would be an amazing experience. When she went there, she said:

> The only labor and delivery I had seen were the birth of my own children ... For someone who is not a physician or nurse or has any medical background it was very exciting.

Susan outlines this first U.S. doula study:

> The first Houston study was a randomized, controlled trial
> of doula support ... One big challenge was finding doulas
> willing to work for what we could afford to pay, and who
> could work unusual hours. If you are a doula with a woman
> in labor, and the labor stretches on, you don't get to go
> home when your 8 hours are done. The way our protocol
> was written, once a doula started with a patient she stayed
> with that patient until the woman delivered. A doula might
> work for over 24 hours with one patient, and then she'd
> need some time off to recover. It was a challenge to enroll
> patients that fit the criteria and to have doulas on call when
> patients came in; but somehow we managed. The main
> result was the decrease in the cesarean rates for women
> who had a doula, an important outcome for the obstetric
> community.

Susan continued:

> When we would present this material, everyone would say,
> "Oh, that's a wonderful finding, but those people didn't
> have family members there."

Of course, the study had been specifically planned that way to test the
benefits of a doula. In truth, the hospital seldom allowed family members to
visit because it was too crowded and there was very little privacy. Curtains
weren't always pulled during an exam or private procedure because people
were always at the bedside and curtains would be in the way. Most women
labored in one big ward with 17 beds arranged in a U-shape around three
sides with a nursing station on the fourth side. If there were too many
women in labor, they would put beds in a walkway. Susan saw at least one
woman deliver in a walkway bed because the baby came so quickly.

The results from Houston I showed the remarkable and significant effects of having a doula for first-time, term mothers with uncomplicated pregnancies. In the final analysis, there were three groups of about 200 women each: a doula group, an observation group, and a control or chart-review group of women who were not actually enrolled in the study, but who met the criteria for enrollment. Cesarean section rates were 8.0% for the doula group, 13.0% for the observed group, and 18.1% for the chart-review group; epidural anesthesia rates for spontaneous vaginal deliveries were 7.8%, 22.6%, and 55.3% respectively; and rates for vaginal deliveries with no medication were 54.7%, 31.3% and 12.3% respectively. There were similar trends for oxytocin use, duration of labor, prolonged infant hospitalization, and maternal fever (Kennell, Klaus, McGrath, Robertson, & Hinkley, 1991).

The Couple's Study in Cleveland

While the concept of a doula had grown out of research in Guatemala, and the proof of principle had been demonstrated in Guatemala and Texas, it was time to further address the concerns of the critics. Families had become more acceptable in U.S. hospitals, and in particular, the baby's father was often present in obstetric units. A continuation of the doula grant was funded to do similar research at the University Hospitals in Cleveland. The study asked whether doulas would still have the same impact if a woman was in labor and her partner was also present. Dr. Kennell describes recruitment:

> We did a large study in 1988 to 1992. The word went out that it was good to get into this family clinic program. As part of the study, we would go to childbirth education classes ... We found it was a gold mine for recruiting patients because everybody was thinking about their baby. It gave us a chance to say something about our plans to study doulas.

Susan explains the two categories of patients:

> Staff patients ... do not have private insurance, so they
> are often covered by Medicare or Medicaid ... Care is
> provided by the staff physician, who would be mostly
> residents working here in the hospital. Private patients
> would be delivered by their private obstetricians, family
> practice doctors, or sometimes, midwives ... In Cleveland,
> at that time, virtually all of the staff patients were African
> American, and the majority of the private patients were
> Caucasian, although certainly not all of them.

Dr. Kennell comments on other differences between the two groups of
patients:

> The private patients had telephones available and were
> used to using them. They would call the study personnel
> or the obstetrician as soon as the first labor pains began.
> We would hear about it quickly because they told the
> person they called that they were in our study and that
> we wanted to know as soon as possible. We enrolled
> almost all the private patients who signed up. We didn't
> draw a randomized slip (control group vs. doula group)
> until patients had been admitted to the hospital. We
> wanted to be sure they were healthy or weren't going to
> be sent home. The staff patients were not used to calling
> doctors and doctors' offices. Many did not have their own
> telephone, and some had their phones disconnected. We
> enrolled a much smaller percentage of the staff patients
> although we had signed up an equal number.

These differences in patient groups created problems for those
analyzing the data because the two types of patients did not give compa-

rable results. The private, middle-class patients showed a significantly lower cesarean rate in the presence of a doula, whether their male partner was there or not. In the smaller group of staff patients, controls showed a somewhat low Cesarean rate for the controls, and there was no significant decrease with a doula.

Due to confounding factors resulting from including both staff and private patients in the study, writing the paper became very complicated. Were the differences racial, socioeconomic, or the experience of the physicians? In addition, staff patients were only about 25% of the patients, and more than half did not have a partner with them. Since these issues detracted from showing the definite positive impact that doulas had among private patients, the investigators did not want to set themselves up for unreasonable criticism. They put the paper aside for a while. In any case, they had already begun the next project: Houston II.

Sometime later, an article on the Cleveland Couples Study was submitted to the journal *Birth*. After looking it over, Michael Klein, of the editorial board, and Diony Young, the editor, together determined that the paper could focus on the larger group of private patients. These patients also more closely fit the study criteria by having a partner present (99%). Susan noted how extremely grateful the authors were for their decision and help. Now the paper could address the 420 middle-class private patients. Three reviewers (neither Diony Young or Michael Klein) all agreed that the study could be accepted with some minor revisions.

Ultimately, in 2008, the study was published. Data showed that patient controls had a 25.0% Cesarean rate while it was 13.4% in the doula group. Significantly fewer women with a doula (64.7%) had epidural analgesia than the control group (76.0%). Also, in a subgroup of women who had induced labor, the Cesarean rate was significantly less for the doula patients (12.5%) than for the control patients (58.8%). On questionnaires, the male partners of women in the doula group were unequivocally positive about receiving doula support (McGrath & Kennell, 2008).

Houston II

Now the investigators planned to examine the effects of a doula versus pain medications. By the time the Cleveland group returned to Houston, Jefferson Davis Hospital had been closed, but another hospital in the same region was available. Ben Taub Hospital served a mostly indigent population, and study patients were 88% Hispanic and 7% African-American. As in all the studies, first-time mothers with low-risk pregnancies were recruited. If there were any complications during the pregnancy, the mother could not be part of the study: no twins, no breech births, no pre-eclampsia, no gestational diabetes, nothing that would label them as high risk, although eliminating pregnancies at high risk did not guarantee a vaginal delivery.

The randomized controlled trial, carried out between 1993 and 1997, had three groups; one group was the epidural group that would receive an epidural at the first indication of pain after a 5 cm cervical dilation; the second group could receive narcotic medication for any indication of pain; and the third group was the doula group. As soon as a woman was enrolled and randomly assigned to the doula group, she could have a doula throughout her labor. Every enrolled woman could receive an epidural or narcotic medication if the medical staff decided the woman needed it. The goal was not to withhold any particular type of medication, but to make sure that a woman wasn't given a particular type of medication as the first choice unless she was assigned to get it based on group membership. There was an additional chart review group that was enrolled after delivery and experienced standard obstetric care.

When Houston II was completed, the investigators obtained amazing results. While the chart-review group had a 26.1% Cesarean rate, the epidural group, a 16.8% rate and the narcotic group, an 11.6% rate, the doula group had a Cesarean rate of 3.1%! The doula group also showed significantly less maternal fever and a lower use of oxytocin and of forceps or vacuum delivery. Susan comments: "To end up with a cesarean rate of

3.1% is remarkable. I don't think you can go much lower than that ... but we can't get the results published!"

A poster was shown at the Society for Research in Child Development on the 531 women (McGrath et al., 1999). The authors sent a full publication to *JAMA*, to *Lancet*, to *NEJM*, and to *Lancet* a second time when they were doing a special issue on women's health, and to *Birth*. Susan continues:

> We're very, very frustrated. *Lancet* and *JAMA* sent it back with no review, saying they weren't interested in the topic at that time. *The New England Journal* wrote a critique of it, down to the font that we used in our paper. (Laughing) OK, it wasn't quite that bad. They questioned absolutely everything. If we were to resubmit it, they wanted such detailed information that it wouldn't fit in their 3000 word limit.

There was a second project on a subgroup of the patients above. Susan explains:

> We did a two month home visit to babies born to mothers in our study, looking at how the mothers interacted with their two-month-old ... The narcotic group and the epidural group were collapsed into a non-doula group ... We found a significant difference. The doula-supported mothers tended to be physically closer to their babies at the home visit; they were more attentive to their babies at two months then the non-doula mothers. We think that's important data, that an intervention that happens only during childbirth, and doesn't continue beyond the first two hours of a baby's life would have an impact on how a mother behaves toward her baby two months later.

Using a quantitative scoring system, the doula mothers tended to be significantly more interactive with their babies than the non-doula mothers on four of five standardized observations. The results for the 104 women were presented at the Society for Research in Child Development in poster format (Landry et al., 1998).

Houston II was no exception to the challenges encountered during clinical studies. Susan tells this story:

> We used to talk with the doula coordinator every single week. We had a scheduled time that Dr. Kennell would talk on the phone with her. If I was in the office that day, we would have a three-way phone conversation. (One time) we received an unexpected phone call from her telling us that we had to stop enrolling patients immediately because the IRB at (Ben Taub) hospital had suddenly without warning taken back their approval ... One of the women on the review board ... had not been involved in the original approval proceedings. She had either just had a baby, or was expecting a baby, and she said, "How can you withhold epidural analgesia from a woman in labor?"... This woman thought every single woman should get an epidural and she thought every woman at this particular hospital did get an epidural ... In fact, we had very carefully set up this study so if a woman in our study wanted an epidural she could get it, no matter which group she was assigned to.

The Cleveland investigators then had to put a lot of data together to present to the review board again. Fortunately, the head of obstetrics at the Houston hospital, Dr. Kenneth Moise, was working with the study, and they could forward the data to him. He successfully described everything to the board and explained that procedures in the study would result in absolutely no damage to the mother or her baby. The study was on hold for a few weeks, but it was a jolt for a study that had been going smoothly.

The Final Cleveland Study

Here, Susan outlines the final study in this series:

> The next doula project was in Cleveland. While we called
> it the Bonding Study, it's as much about doulas as it is
> about bonding. We also called it the Evolutionary Model
> of Childbirth. The idea is that laboring with the support
> of another woman, and having your baby with you and
> placed immediately with you right after you give birth, and
> keeping your baby right by your side for the first 24 or
> 48 hours, was closer to the way childbirth had happened
> for eons. Now for the past 110 years or so, a mother's
> labor and delivery takes place in a hospital surrounded
> by medical personnel rather then family members, often
> with the mother being anesthetized and only seeing the
> baby after it's all cleaned up.
>
> Thanks to Dr. Kennell and Dr. Klaus, we can now keep
> our babies in the room with us while we're in the hospital,
> but not too many women get their baby placed on them
> immediately after birth. If they are placed there, it's usually
> just for a minute or so before the baby is whisked away to
> have procedures done: they are put under a warmer so
> they can be weighed and measured, get vitamin K, eye
> drops, and so on. Then they're usually brought back to
> the mother all bundled up, like a little package.
>
> In our Evolutionary Model of childbirth, we believe that
> the baby should be delivered and placed on the mother's
> abdomen, skin to skin. The baby might be wiped off with
> some towels so he or she wouldn't be quite so slippery,
> but then the mother and baby would be left like that for

up to two hours or until the first breastfeeding occurred. With the baby making his or her way, basically unaided, up to the mother's breast we'd let the baby decide when to begin the first feeding.

Between July 1998 and June 2004, we enrolled 363 women in the project, with 287 completing the study. There were three groups randomly assigned. The first group was the control group. They would receive all the standard care, just as it was given here at MacDonald hospital. The second group would have a doula with them from the beginning to the end of their labor and delivery. The doula would stay for the first two hours after delivery and encourage and support self-attachment and a skin-to-skin position for the mother and baby. Self-attachment means attachment of the baby to the nipple, not the mother and baby being bonded or that kind of attachment. The third group was exactly like the second group, except there was an additional meeting with the doula during which she would encourage the mother to carry her baby as much as possible in the first two months. The mother would be given a soft sling-like carrier to make carrying easier (Ainsfield, Casper, Nozyce, & Cunningham, 1990). Basically, the mother was being asked to have her baby on her body as much as possible in those first two months.

The final outcome measure for this study was different from what we had done in the past. As before we kept all of the perinatal data: the kind and length of delivery, the kind of anesthesia, the baby's Apgar scores, did the mother initiate breastfeeding or was she going to bottle feed, etc. But we also had all the mothers bring their baby to our office when the baby was about 14-months-old to do the Ainsworth Strange Situation. That is a very specific test to look at the health of the baby's attachment to his or her mother, not the bonding of the mother to the baby. Mary Ainsworth hypothesized that all babies are attached to their mother, but some babies are securely attached and other babies are insecurely attached. A securely attached infant will grow up to be an emotionally and mentally healthy adult with good adult relationships and positive parenting skills. An insecurely attached infant will be more likely to grow up with psychological problems—anxiety, depression, and poor relationships with adults and then become a poorer parent.

Our hypothesis was that a mother having a doula present during labor and delivery would be the kind of parent who would be more sensitive, more empathic, and more tuned into her baby's needs. This would more likely result in a securely attached infant at 14 months. What are our results? We don't know because we have 287 videotapes that still need to be scored for attachment. Scoring requires a two week training by the Ainsworth experts at the University of Minnesota. There is no money to pay someone at least $100 per tape--it takes a minimum of two hours to score each tape. So that's where the study stands.

Note: John Kennell quotations were taken from an unpublished interview conducted by Mary Hellerstein, MD on August 23, 2007 and from the 1995 SCRD Oral History Interview by Susan McGrath. Susan McGrath quotations were taken from unpublished interviews conducted by Mary Hellerstein, M.D. on September 27, 2007 and March 12, 2008.

A COMPASSIONATE CAREER LIVES ON

John Kennell died on August 27, 2013, at age 91. He had gone to his office daily until November, 2011. At his 90th birthday party on January 9, 2012, he enjoyed dancing with his beloved wife, Peggy, and socializing with his colleagues in the division of developmental behavioral pediatrics at Case Western Reserve University (See Photo).

John Kennell left an extraordinary legacy. Come what may, he kept proposing solutions that were often considered messy or inconvenient—family members underfoot in the labor ward and hospital rooms, or a doula in the delivery suite. He was not the only one pushing for a more caring health system for children and their parents, but he stands out in the minds of many for promoting positive change, pursuing difficult research, and inspiring others to do the same.

A charming account about John Kennell was written by Sandra B. Erlanger in the 1991 November CWRU magazine. She wrote,

> It really is phenomenal that a human relationship has a
> more powerful effect on the outcome of labor than all
> the methods available in obstetrics. Doulas are a great

godsend for fathers as well as mothers. The doula takes the heavy burden of the mother's well being off the father's shoulders so he can be attentive, affectionate and supportive.

Erlanger noted another important aspect:

Studies performed as a result of the work of Drs. Kennell and Klaus showed that the help of a doula has the greatest impact on economically disadvantaged, unsupported mothers.

The 1970s and 1980s represented a golden age for the neonatologists, pediatricians, and others instigating for change in hospital policies in order to make it possible for families to join mothers and newborns in the hospital. Changes from one part of the U.S. spread rapidly to other areas, and many of the changes are still in place. However, increasing technological advances sometimes interfered. Dr. Kennell commented in 1995,

As obstetrics has become more technical and more interventionist, the nurses have been under greater pressure to do all sorts of other things than staying with the mother ... Both neonatology and obstetrics are determined to find the one baby in a thousand that might have trouble, leading the other 999 babies and their parents to have a more stressful experience than would be desirable. Now there is a much greater need for a doula than a few years ago.

Susan McGrath, Dr. Kennell's longtime research partner said,

The significance of the doula is that mothers who have a doula are much more positive about the birthing experience itself, more positive about their partners, and more positive about their baby.

She noted that the research is not so accepted by the medical community because it's "low tech."

> There's no fancy machine, no medication, no clever procedure. It's based on something so intuitive, and so old-fashioned, that it isn't seen as important ... unless you happen to be the woman in labor who doesn't have a doula. Then you realize how important it is to have someone there, just for you. You need the medical people who are looking out for the medical well being of the mother and baby. In addition you need someone there to focus on the emotional well being of a woman who is about to face one of the most emotional moments of her life—meeting her baby for the first time .... Dr. Kennell and I believe that experiences during labor and in the first minutes, hours and days after a baby is born have a deep impact. The reassuring presence of a doula may not only change how the woman mothers her baby in the first hours or days, but how the child ends up as an adult.

McGrath continued, "Despite our very nice results, they are not about the life-and-death topics that attract funding, such as curing cancer or eliminating AIDS. A long-term study would be a tremendous challenge, but we think it would be worth it. How do you get the funding for it? That's tough."

Still, good ideas about doulas have taken root. Training and practice for doulas has been beautifully and comprehensively described in *The Doula Book* (Klaus et al., 2002, 2012). There is also a professional organization of doulas established in 1991: DONA International (www.dona.com). John Kennell was one of the founders.

Doula advocates include Irving Harris (1910-2005), an entrepreneur in Chicago, who was an avid supporter of Doula programs for families, and encouraged others to financially support them. He felt it was vital to understand the role of culture and community in childbearing and childrearing decisions. Most women, even those who do not receive adequate prenatal care, know that prenatal care is important to healthy pregnancy outcomes. Those who bottle-feed know that breast-feeding is better for an infant's health. Simply knowing these facts, however, does not seem enough to persuade a mother to make informed birth choices. One of the most difficult things they had in the Beethoven Project, from the beginning, was trying to teach women who didn't want to learn how they should care for babies. So the wonderful thing about the doula program was it seemed to reach the young mother when she was most able to hear—when she wanted to learn about her labor: how difficult it was going to be, how long it was going to last. When the doula offered to be with her every minute throughout the labor and help her with all the problems, the woman appreciated it.

The program Irving Harris supported reinforced the findings of Kennell and Klaus. Harris said,

> Doula programs piloted by the collaborative Chicago Doula Project have achieved significant success by ... integrating the doula model of perinatal support into team support in three very different community agencies. It's absolutely wonderful what the doulas have done. Rates of adequate prenatal care have risen. Birth outcomes have improved. Both cesarean and epidural rates were reduced and breastfeeding increased dramatically ... Additionally, mothers feel empowered by their birth and breastfeeding experiences, and are more equipped to advocate for themselves and for their babies. The teens served by the project are talking to their babies more, touching them more, and interacting with them more. Our program has further demonstrated that community based doulas can contribute in profoundly

significant ways to help people surmount socio-cultural barriers and have healthy birth outcomes.

Harris also commented that the doula paraprofessionals they trained were paid about the same as home visitors, still a relatively low price compared to nurses. He's heard new doulas say at graduation time, "I never in all my life thought I'd ever have a job like this, the opportunity to really make a difference. It's wonderful." Known as HealthConnect One, the Doula program remains a community force in Chicago (2014).

Continuing Global Legacy

Kennell was a leader in global child health education, urging the American Academy of Pediatrics to develop global child health programs in the 80s. He served on the first task force to begin that process. He was also a member of the Standing Committee of the International Pediatric Association in the 90s. For 22 years, he was a board member of Health Frontiers, an organization that planned and implemented the first postgraduate medical training in Laos.

Kennell believed that American medical students should have knowledge and skills related to global child health and cross-cultural differences. For 18 years, he taught in a CWRU seminar series, "Preparation for International Service," for medical students, nursing students and residents. He discussed all he had learned about caring for infants in Guatemalan villages. He also taught for 12 years in the annual CWRU workshop on "Management of disasters: focus on children and families," where he explained how children perceive death at different developmental stages, and how to help bereaved children. Colleagues who are still teaching in these courses continue to reflect the teaching legacy of Dr. Kennell.

Continuing Student Legacy

In his later years, John Kennell's wisdom continued to inspire students in the United States and abroad. For example, Dr. Niramol Patjanasoontorn, a child psychiatrist from Thailand, came to Cleveland in 1996 to accompany her husband who was doing a fellowship at University Hospitals.

When John Kennell called to offer her a position as a fellow in developmental behavioral pediatrics, she literally jumped with joy, surprising her two young daughters. When she began her studies with Kennell she reports,

> I saw many books in his room that I had never seen before—on attachment theory, natural birth with a doula, and child development—too many to list. I began to read them and to watch study guide videos. Truly, Dr. Kennell's character and his devotion to the attachment of mother and child inspired me.

Dr. Niramol said that Dr. Kennell would be pleased to know that she put a lecture on "Attachment in Infants" into the medical student curriculum for the first time in her Thai university.

Another physician, Denise Bothe, first met John Kennell when interviewing for a fellowship in developmental behavioral pediatrics. His interest in international health, and research on infant mother bonding was a great inspiration for her. Dr. Bothe said,

> When he would teach, he clearly had a wealth of wisdom. One of his early teachings about research was to tell me that one of the most important things for a researcher is to take long walks in the park to think. I know he is right about that, and it is true in my life that those times are when the creative ideas come into my head. I treasure his wisdom because I knew how successful he was at

focusing his life's work on such important topics. Every time I heard him lecture about his research in Guatemala, I learned more. He had so much knowledge, and the more I heard him talk, the more I learned about what is really important in life. He is such a sweet, humble, and caring person, and always interested in listening to what I had to say. With our offices so close, we had the opportunity for many thoughtful conversations about research, or just life. He always treated me and any one else with whom I saw him interact as an equal, and that was also a great example for me. I am so grateful to have known such a great man. I have also been honored to know his wife Peggy, and am inspired by their long marriage and commitment to each other.

Dr. Bothe is now a faculty member in the division of developmental behavioral pediatrics at Case Western Reserve University.

Changes Now Taken for Granted

Starting about 40 years ago in the United States, family members were allowed, for the first time, to be present with mothers in labor in hospitals. Following delivery, infants were allowed to room with their mothers. Fathers and siblings were allowed to visit the new member of their family. Millions of families have lived this now expected and normal experience. Young parents have most likely not heard of John Kennell, the gentle, compassionate, courageous pediatrician who came to believe that they should be together with each other and their new baby during these important life events. They can't imagine that things were ever different!

John Kennell deserves gratitude from families in the U.S. and around the world for his leadership in emphasizing the importance of early mother-infant attachment, in promoting generous parental visitation for hospitalized children, for documenting the grief that parents of newborns suffer and pioneering bereavement groups for them, for facilitating child life programs in hospitals and for documenting the value of doulas in supporting mothers through labor. Now it is up to his students to carry on!

Note: John Kennell quotations were taken from an unpublished interview conducted by Mary Hellerstein, MD on August 23, 2007, and from the 1995 SCRD Oral History Interview by Susan McGrath. Susan McGrath quotations were taken from unpublished interviews conducted by Mary Hellerstein, M.D. on September 27, 2007 and March 12, 2008.

SECTION III

TRIBUTES

T. BERRY BRAZELTON, MD

Sixty years ago, John and I were in a pediatric residency at the Children's Hospital in Boston. He was an extraordinary person then, and it was easy to predict that he was headed for leadership in Pediatrics. At a time when many interns and residents were recovering from the aftermath of World War II, he stood out as a bright, kind, generous, and effective resident. We all loved him. Most of our colleagues were fighting their way up the ladder at Children's and Harvard, for that was the rule. John offered a hand to help others up the ladder. Unique and wonderful. Our leader and professor, Charlie Janeway, was like that. But not many were at Harvard.

We used to talk a lot about how to help parents rear their children, how stressful it must be, how labor, delivery, and the new baby was such a vulnerable time for parents—but had become so medicalized that parents were stripped of any controls and, if their passion for the new baby survived, it was a miracle. We were led in our psychological thinking by Dane Prugh and Helen Glazer, but it was not a popular era for pediatric training in those days (or now). Children's in Boston was thought to be a residency for training specialists (cardiology, neurology, anesthesia, NICU, immunology, even cancer), and all our efforts were to be devoted to those areas. None of us were expected to become general pediatricians, or as we have, behavioral pediatricians. For example, when I turned down Janeway's chief residency for child psychiatry, he said, "And waste all this good pediatric training!" But in 1990, when I did a rapid survey of pediatric graduates from CHMC, 80%

had gone into practice and general pediatrics. Only 20% had become the specialists we were being trained for. And the 80% had had little exposure to child development, making relationships with parents to further the child's development, or anything related to infant mental health. This is to emphasize that John Kennell's path has been in spite of his training. His own bony nose has pointed him toward the elegant paths he has taken—in teaching, research, and advocacy. He is a hero.

I watched him woo and capture his first and permanent wife, Peggy. She was the head surgical nurse for Dr. Robert Gross, our most famous cardiac surgeon. John was brave and successful in that area, too. It was both fun and frightening to see the feelings he stirred up in the hospital. All the pediatric nurses had been stationing themselves in his path, for he was such a lovely, outstanding man. All were terribly disappointed in his choice. The surgical floors were rabid at her defection when Peggy decided to marry him and leave them. So, I have known and loved John and Peggy for a long, long time. We have almost circled the world with our advocacy and our teaching. My Neonatal Behavioral Assessment was first published in 1973, at about the same time as John and Marshall Klaus "hit the fan" with their wonderful ideas and research about the opportunity right after birth for enhancing a parent's passionate attachment to the neonate.

Their early papers recommended that the birth process be de-medicalized so the new mother could both participate and be alert for her baby immediately after birth in order to attach. Grantly Dick Read of England and Lamaze from France had advocated that we discontinue premedication for women so they could be awake for labor and delivery. In 1961, I had published a paper on the effects of "twilight sleep," which was in common-usage for mothers-to-be, to tide them through labor painlessly. It was a combination of 75 mg Demerol, 200 mg phenobarbital, and 25 mg of atropine. These babies had satisfactory Apgars at birth, probably in response to labor and the stimuli of the new environment. In the newborn nursery, for at least 2 days thereafter, the nurses reported having to watch the babies for aspiration and choking on their mucous. By observation, these neonates were depressed and difficult to rouse. For, when the cord was cut, the neonate was left with the mother's circulating level of drugs. With an immature liver for detoxification, and with immature kidneys for secretion, an immature and more vulnerable brain, we found that the newborn was behaviorally less responsive for 5 to 7 days after birth. We postulated that they would be less open to maternal attachment efforts if their mothers had been pre-medicated for labor and delivery.

With the urgent cry from Klaus and Kennell in the mid-sixties to have the baby ready after birth for attachment to the new mother, our work had a powerful effect on the obstetrical practices. I remember a delivery at the Boston Lying-In by Dr. Arthur Gorbach, one of our more *avant garde* obstetricians. He was trying to follow the Lamaze recommendation to deliver a non-medicated mother: a quiet supportive labor and delivery room, and sharing the new baby with the mother right after birth, to attach as recommended by Klaus and Kennell. All through labor and delivery, he shushed nurses and observers. The baby was delivered easily and successfully, cried out dutifully to make the first sound in the quiet delivery room. He shushed the baby, but to no avail. He handed the crying baby to the mother, who immediately cuddled her baby and he quieted. She even put the new baby to her breast to suckle. The newborn responded eagerly. At this point, the nurses took the baby away from her, washed off the vernix, and swaddled the now screaming infant. They rushed him off to the neonatal nursery, leaving the new mother and father empty handed and open-mouthed. The procedure had been followed, but it would be several more years before Klaus and Kennell's work would really be incorporated. But we were on our way.

Marshall, John, and I lectured around the country at the behest of every Childbirth Education Association site. We urged parents to fight for changes in the delivery system in America. We started up groups of faithful followers. They were members of the "choir." They believed, as we did, that labor and delivery should be at the choice of the patient. Women who wanted to learn how to labor from childbirth education groups should be respected and valued. To be awake to greet your new baby was an attainable, magnificent goal.

In the United States middle-classes, our encouragement prevailed, for they were able to fight for the kind of labor and delivery we recommended. Middle-class delivery hospitals began to change. Underserved poor, less fortunate parents still have to endure medicated deliveries and more old fashioned practices of separation from their babies in many hospitals. In other hospitals, the changes Kennell and Klaus recommended have affected all classes!

I lectured about the competence of the newborn and how powerful his behavior could be when it was shared with new parents. It was a bridge for them to see him as a person, and to feel that they could begin to see their way as new parents. Klaus lectured on the importance of bonding and its ultimate enhancement of permanent attachment between parents and the baby. We were popular as a duo.

One night, after weeks of lecturing together, I said to Marshall, "I can't stand to give this lecture one more time." He answered, "I can't stand to hear it. I tell you what, you give mine and I'll give yours." We did, and it worked. Hospitals that were in the *avant garde* movement we were fighting for began to place signs on new parents' doors—"No entry. Parents bonding."

We were being successful in starting to take away the birth process from insensitive medical practices. It created anger and hostility in many of our profession. One professor at Harvard said, "You've ruined my life. I worked all my professional life to be sure women were anesthetized during labor. Otherwise, they're like animals and I can't stand it! You just want them to suffer."

John and Marshall were criticized for their emphasis on the importance of the time immediately after birth as critical for reinforcing the process of attachment. Bowlby and Ainsworth had brought the concept of parent-infant attachment to the surface as a critical base for the future of the baby's optimal development. Attachment would occur best when the passion of the mother (the parents) was at its peak, right after delivery. The criticism of the infant researchers who could not tolerate the "critical" or "sensitive" period right after delivery was aimed at John Kennell and Marshall Klaus. It hurt them at the time. I had been through criticisms about my neonatal assessment scale, so I could reassure them that it was professional jealousy. I think this criticism turned them to study a new area—the "doula" concept.

What great clinicians and researchers they have been!

In 1968, my wife and I spent a summer on the island off Thera (Santorini) in Greece. It is the rim of the volcano whose eruption covered Crete and had just been found that year, as airplane observers spotted the square stones of the walls underwater on the coast of Thera. They realized that square stones were manmade and began to uncover the extensive ruins of a Minoan 15th century B.C. they called "the Lost Atlantis." Professor Emily Vermuele, Professor of Antiquities from Harvard was asked (as the only American) to help uncover this city. She had small children, and asked me and my wife to accompany her as their pediatrician to this small island off Thera. There were no physicians on this island.

We were bored with digging and began to accompany the one midwife to deliver babies. We had a fascinating experience. A woman in labor was given tin cans and old bottles to throw at her husband, who groaned for her with each labor pain. "It is my job," he said.

When the baby was delivered, I was used to rushing up to the mother so she could "bond," as John and Marshall had suggested. These Greek ladies would say, "Not yet" and turn toward the wall. After 30 minutes or so, they'd recover their own resources, turn back to say, "Now I want my baby." Their bonding followed their own recovery. The critical period was postponed. I reported this to John and Marshall. We could see that the critical period they had recommended was culture bound. Their recommendations had been in the United States culture, where the medical teams had taken away a natural process. In order to overcome this, mothers should be allowed to be rewarded with their newborn right away—maybe before they had recovered themselves. But their work had sunk a wedge into the medicalized delivery and postnatal hospital custom. Mothers were respected for wanting their babies nearby, and were even encouraged to have time for "bonding" each day. Most services have changed dramatically as a result of the early research and writing of John Kennell and Marshall Klaus.

The research that Kennell and Klaus turned to in establishing the value of a "doula," a female accompanist to a woman in labor, has been just as powerful. They were sensitive to the possibility of losing the father-to-be as a companion for his laboring wife, so they demonstrated that the effects of having a doula present was an addition to the importance of having her significant other—the father—to encourage and advise a woman in labor.

The powerful effects of a doula as a companion are changing many hospitals, and will have more and more influence in making labor and delivery a well-supported humane process in which both the new mother and father will feel valued, respected, and powerful in this step toward bonding to their new offspring. The passion which is generated and builds up in the nine months of pregnancy deserves to be enhanced and celebrated by a successful and psychologically healthy delivery to enhance the attachment between the parents and their infant, as well as between themselves. Their work has been a beacon of light and hope for families who are under more stress than they can handle in our present world.

WILLIAM B. CAREY, MD

I t is a great honor and pleasure for me to write this tribute to my colleague and old friend, John Kennell. I have known him for many years, and am one of his most ardent fans. Since I first heard of and met him, we have shared some important experiences.

I first learned of him in the early 1960s by way of his paper in *Pediatrics* about the emotional significance of the newborn period. My behavioral mentors at CHOP at that time made sure that I was aware that this man knew what he was talking about and should be heeded.

I did not meet him until several years later, probably in 1969, at an Academy of Pediatrics meeting, when he was introducing some of his important work about parent-infant relations in the newborn period. He was also quite supportive of my first presentation at that same session of my heretical notions about innate differences of temperament in children.

A long and cordial relationship has followed. I recall in particular two significant experiences we have shared, one pleasant and the other more tempestuous. The first was that in those early days, the Academy met frequently in Chicago at the Palmer House, which was conveniently located only a short distance from the splendid Chicago Art Institute. I forget how many times it happened, but I can recall finding him over there repeatedly during meetings when we were supposed to be paying close attention to the latest developments in pediatrics nearby. He was observing with great interest the paintings of the Madonna and child, mostly the medieval ones, noting how Mary was holding her baby, and whether they were facing each other or not, as portrayed by artists like Giotto and his contemporaries. I was more interested in the glorious Renaissance depiction of mothers and their babies by later masters like Botticelli. John was concentrating more on the relationships as expressed by physical positioning. I was admiring the advanced, elegant technique and the feeling depicted. We ran into each other where the earlier period evolved into the later. My guess is that we learned as much about development from these diversions as did our somnolent colleagues in the stuffy conference rooms. Our friendship was established. Since then, we have enjoyed together a number of similar displays at such places as the Gardner Museum in Boston.

We also shared the similar, but less joyful experience of being scorned by our colleagues for our unorthodox ideas about human nature and child development, which ran contrary to the received wisdom of the times; his advancing his recognition of the great psychological importance to parents of the earliest hours and days of their child's life; my reporting findings about the compelling evidence for largely inborn, clinically significant temperament traits.

John Kennell, the observant clinician, could see plainly that in these beginnings of life, mothers needed to be together with their newborns and with other members of their families, not separated by bacterially and emotionally sterile barriers, as was the accepted practice when he and I were trained, and which still prevailed then. His conviction was based on extensive clinical observations. There was considerable public enthusiasm for his view, but also widespread and often derogatory professional resistance. Also, unfortunately, some overly enthusiastic people exaggerated the concept of parent-infant bonding, and misapplied it. John and Marshall Klaus had to endure these and other unfavorable reactions. However, it is beyond dispute that they made an enormous contribution to humanizing neonatal pediatrics. The vast differences between the nurseries of our early years, and those of the present, are surely largely a result of their experience, wisdom, and courage. Their clinical observations in a variety of settings informed them that they were right and that they should not let the critics dissuade them.

My experience with being scorned was somewhat similar. It is hard to believe now, in the aftermath of the Decade of the Brain, but in the 1950s and 1960s, all variations and deviations of behavior were widely believed to be due exclusively to the imprint of the environment. Nothing was thought to be innate except some forms of mental retardation. Following the creative lead of Stella Chess, Alexander Thomas, and their group in the New York Longitudinal Study, I began to develop a series of parent questionnaires to facilitate the clinical elaboration of their nine largely inborn behavioral style traits. I did this at first by myself, but soon was joined by some bright young graduate students in psychology at Temple University in Philadelphia. Over the span of about 15 years, we produced five different psychometrically competent scales for various ages from one month to 12 years. The response of our colleagues to these efforts was a mixture of ignoring, praising, and criticizing them for various reasons. Some critics argued that these traits did not exist, but were just being imagined by the mothers; others asserted that they might exist, but one could not trust mothers to report them adequately; and others assured us that they did not matter anyway. The clumsiness of some of the complaints from certain members of the establishment was remarkable. The most confident rejections seemed to come from childless academics.

Why is it that some who claim to be scientists are often so resistant to scientific evidence, such as was offered by John Kennell and me? To my surprise, I found an answer in the first canto of the *Divine Comedy*, where Dante describes his midlife crisis, when he cannot reach the joyful mountain of knowledge. His progress is impeded by three beasts; the lion, the wolf, and the leopard, thought by scholars to stand for pride, avarice, and lust or lack of restraint. It seemed to me that the three beasts could be readily transposed into the scientific field as representing respectively; the lion—the conservative forces of resistance to novelty; the wolf—the spoilers who attack ideas for personal rather than scientific reasons; and the leopard—the opportunists who misuse new ideas for their own purposes rather than for the advancement of knowledge or human well-being. John and I had to contend with all three kinds of beasts. My conclusion in my review was that we must train ourselves to recognize the beasts for what they are, defend ourselves as best we can, and keep on marching through the dark forest toward the mountain of knowledge (*J Dev Beh Pediat.* 14: 53-56, 1993).

As John and I continue to march on, I feel for him a strong affection for his friendship and great admiration for his work. Dante suggested that help in this struggle with the beasts might come from the greyhound, who would bring with him / her the qualities of wisdom, love, and virtue. I especially salute John Kennell for his embodiment of these qualities.

The Children's Hospital of Philadelphia
December 12, 2007

DALIA ZEMAITYTE

All material below is from an interview with Dalia Zemaityte and John Kennell on 5/31/2007. They were colleagues and friends for more than 50 years at Rainbow Babies and Children's Hospital.

Dalia's Early Life

Dalia was born in Siaulai, Lithuania. Her father was the Dean of the School of Veterinary Medicine in the capitol, and was professor of surgery part of the time. In the summer, she would go to visit her uncle in the country. But in 1944, when the war broke out, she couldn't go back to her family. At that time, the Russians were advancing and the Germans were retreating. Dalia's uncle and many other Lithuanians went to Germany to escape Communism. Unfortunately, her parents didn't know this and wouldn't leave without Dalia. She never saw them again because she went directly to the United States from Germany in 1948. In Germany, Dalia was classified as an orphan and didn't have to wait for a visa to the United States. When she informed the American Embassy in Frankfort that she did not want to go, they could not believe it. Even though her uncle and his family had to wait for visas they said, "You just go, it's an opportunity." Her parents were killed under unknown circumstances in 1957. After restrictions were lifted, the first time Dalia could go back was 1972. Now she visits Lithuania every year.

Dalia finished high school in Yonkers and completed her baccalaureate in nursing education in Syracuse. Then in 1958, she came to Cleveland's Frances Payne Bolton School of nursing for her Master's degree in nursing administration. While Dalia wished to return to her beloved Syracuse, Olga Benderoff, the director of nursing at Babies and Children's offered a position as a supervisor there. She liked the director so much that she said, "Yes, I'll stay a year." Dalia stayed—more than 50 years.

Working at RB&C

I really loved Babies and Children's. I loved people I worked with and that's where I met John Kennell. I thought we just had a wonderful culture at Babies and Children's. I had never been in a position where the physicians and nurses worked as colleagues and partners, and to me that was very important. Bill Wallace was the chief of staff when I arrived. I came to know John Kennell because as nursing supervisor, I went to all the divisions. We had a preemie suite—now called neonatal intensive care, and John was one of the neonatologists.

At that time, Bowlby and Robertson in England had shown movies and written a book about how depressed hospitalized children are if they are not visited. We started to think about how important families are, and we were one of the first hospitals to understand that parents play an important role in the care of children. John and Marshall were instrumental in allowing longer visiting hours. The hardest thing was to convince physicians and nurses that parents have the right to be with their children. They thought parents were going to be underfoot all the time, asking questions. I said, "It's not our child, it's their child." John was very supportive.

It was a struggle when I think back, but little by little we extended visiting hours. Finally we had unlimited visiting hours and then encouraged parents to participate in care. It's not magical to come to the hospital and feed the baby because they feed them at home. Somehow we thought that aspect was for medical staff. I felt strongly that our culture needed to think that families are essential in the care of children, and this blossomed and continues to blossom. Yet without the support of select medical staff, this would not have happened.

For John and I, meeting Dr. Brazelton was especially helpful. Dr. Brazelton was in the Association for Care of Children's Health. It was a group that was instrumental in stressing the concept of bringing disciplines together including parents for the best of the child. Emma Plank was extremely helpful and got me involved in that association. I was considered one of the founding members but she was truly a founding member. There I learned so much about families and cooperation and partnership. John attended some of the meetings too. It was around for about 20 years and served a very good purpose. The national organization disappeared about 10 to 15 years ago. I really miss it because I thought it was a really interdisciplinary group. Still I think the seeds were sown and many organizations picked up from there and moved on. Even child life came into existence in those days, and then it branched off and had its own group. Nursing had its own organization.

Now there is the Institute for Family Centered Care that also does a lot with family involvement. We belong to it because I felt it was important. We started the Family Advisory Council in 1991. Everything we do in the hospital is looked at through the parents' eyes and it has been a wonderful group. They helped us with building Horvitz Tower. The parents went with different staff to different hospitals. They selected the best features that were then incorporated into Horvitz Tower. For example, the parents helped us write the Patient's Bill of Rights. Now they are helping us with emergency room features because we are planning to build a new emergency room. How you and I see it is not how parents see it. The parent's perspective is very important. This all started back in the early 60s with the culture at Babies and Children's, and it continues to develop.

I remember when we had infants on the first floor at Babies and Children's. Everybody wore isolation gowns, parents and staff. I remember coming out of school full of energy in the 1960s. I said, "We don't need to wear gowns, just have good hand washing." You should have seen the uproar. I think John was the one supporting me. Basically people would wear a gown, but wouldn't wear it the right way, inside out. So we took the gowns off. That was a revolution. I think guidelines are better than rules: when you have a rule you don't have to think. Maybe for one child it's okay to have 3 people at the bedside, but for another family maybe one at the bedside is best. So you have to think about each family and their situation and use the best judgment you can to fulfill the needs of the family. I forever bend the rules. My favorite saying is, "Don't ask for permission ask for forgiveness." If you ask for permission you would never accomplish anything because you will always have somebody say it won't work. If it doesn't you change and move on.

I really love RBC. People come and go, but there is always a core of people that stay. To me the culture is always more important than strategy. You can have all kinds of strategy, but if you don't have a culture to support it, it won't work. People are going to come and do their thing, but they may not be part of the culture. It's not a job, it's a culture you work in. Either people support that or they don't. I was reading the book by Frank Lee who used to be a hospital administrator (not at RB&C). The title is, *If Disney Ran Your Hospital*. It really shows the culture at Disney and what a difference it makes. For example, they show job applicants a movie of what Disney is all about and how they expect you to behave and dress. They call you cast players, not employees. They show you it's more than a job. It's interesting that about 15% of applicants who watch that movie never put their application in. I wonder what would happen if we did that at RB&C. People could say this is not for me. I can't be courteous all the time. I can't smile all the time. I can't put myself in somebody else's shoes and comfort them. That's what I mean about culture. At RB&C, it's because of what we are and what we believe in.

I never called parents visitors. They are parents. I always say there is a distinction between visitors and family. For visitors, we have guidelines for visiting, but for parents we don't. They can come anytime and stay with their child as much as they can. That's why our whole Horvitz Tower was built with private rooms so our parents could stay. Even in our cramped quarters before the Tower was built, parents stayed overnight. They sat on reclining chairs and we had cots. I'll never forget one mom who came with a sleeping bag and said "I'm not going to take up any room," and she stayed under the crib. It makes you think how cruel we had been, not allowing parents to stay with their children. You and I as adults need someone to support us when we're staying in the hospital. If rules were made to prevent infection, I think staff caused more infection than the parents did by not washing hands and going from place to place. Now we send children home with parents doing broviac care. We thought we were the only ones that could do it!

I never did direct care in the preemie suite. I facilitated what was to be done, but did not take care of patients. One day a head nurse came to me and said, "Dalia, I have to ask you something." The husband of one of her nurses was mowing the lawn and found baby rabbits, but the mother had been killed. So the nurse had brought in six baby rabbits. We put them into incubators and I made a schedule. We fed them by pipette because they were so tiny. Whenever someone came to visit we would throw blankets over the incubator. They all survived. It was wonderful. There was a storage room where we kept extra incubators, so we raised those bunnies. Now people would go totally bananas.

John has been helpful with the Family Centered Care Award that is given to the staff at Rainbow Babies & Children's. He has always been an integral part, helping us look at nominations and selecting the recipient. Any physician, nurse, housekeeping person: whoever exhibits the criteria for family-centered care can receive the reward.

I never met anybody so kind and humble at the same time, a truly exceptional human being. John always has a smile. It just makes you feel so good to be in his presence. I love the man. John's influence made the difference in recognizing the importance of parents in the care of their child in the clinical setting. I know this from personal experience. John and Marshall did so much for our babies in the premature suite. Also there was Jane Cable, a head nurse who worked very closely with John. She died maybe 5 or 6 years ago. She was a wonderful person who taught me a lot. She mentored nurses who became really outstanding.

SUSAN MCGRATH AND
HER EXPERIENCES WITH
DR. KENNELL

In the previous chapter on doula research, Susan McGrath has given us many insights about Dr. Kennell's work. But there is more we can learn from her about the man himself. Here's how they met for the first time.

> He came to the door of my hospital room at MacDonald Hospital the day after my 2nd son was born, April 24th, 1984. He stood very politely at the door. He was wearing a white coat and looking very doctor-like; he had a tie on. I had no idea who he was and he knocked on the door and asked if I was Susan McGrath. And I said, yes. I assumed he was some doctor checking up on me the day after the baby was born, or else he had some news about my baby. Then he told me who he was and wanted to know if I was interested in a job! That made me pull up the neckline of my hospital gown and try to look a little more professional than a woman who had just given birth 24 hours before.
>
> This story really goes back to Dr. Kennell and his wonderful networking. He's a man who establishes and maintains relationships with people. He's the kind of person who always sends a thank you letter. He calls people and thanks

them. He's a believer in face-to-face interaction. He hand delivers something that could be sent through campus mail so he would get a chance to talk to the person to maintain a relationship. Networking is really how he got me. He knew the person who had been my research advisor when I was a graduate student. That's how he knew who I was and how to get in touch with me. He called and found, "Oh, she's having a baby," and he tracked me down to that hospital room. I think that was pretty impressive.

I took the job because it was convenient. It was part-time, with flexible hours. I had been working a more structured position as a clinical psychologist in an agency in Lake County. I knew I couldn't go back to that job and juggle a 3-year-old, a newborn, and a husband with challenging work hours from January to April. I had a fair amount of research experience, and had worked with Maureen Hack on her preemie follow-ups. I knew quite a bit about preemies from reading, not from hands-on. I had done a lot of follow-up testing and knew a lot about medical complications, so I wasn't new to the medical arena.

The job seemed like a good fit with my experience and what I liked to do. Dr. Kennell seemed like a nice enough person. I also knew his work with bonding and thought it was important, but didn't know anything about doulas. So the job was convenient—then I got hooked! I can't tell you when or how that happened.

I've worked with Dr. Kennell for 23 years, and still call him Dr. Kennell. I think of him as a friend, and I know he's told me to call him John, but Dr. Kennell seemed right to me because of his experience and professional attitude and age and all the respect I have for him. He's just always been Dr. Kennell to me.

Conversations with Dr Kennell

There have been times we'd be together in the office three-to-four times per week. Other times, I might not see him for a couple weeks, depending on what grant we were working on and how much money there was to pay people. We've also talked about almost every topic under the sun. We are both big Cleveland sports fans, so we'd talk about the Cleveland Indians and the Cleveland Browns. Did you hear the game yesterday? Did you watch the game? We would commiserate about problems of certain players or what the manager was doing. We always had that in common. We'd talk about various TV shows and radio programs, usually NPR and PBS. I'd share things that I'd hear on NPR with him, and he might share a PBS television show he saw that was interesting or worthwhile with me. We'd come in and joke about the various sketches we saw on Saturday Night Live. Our conversations covered everything from the totally intellectual to the most ridiculous.

Dr. Kennell has always been interested in my family. He probably knows more about my children, and their development, and their accomplishments than even my own extended family know. He always took pride in anything I told him about my kids. I loved to share with him all the good things my kids were doing. Then he did the same with his own family. I've heard him talk about his children and their spouses and partners; and his grandchildren. He is so proud of all of them. If they've had any problems, he certainly has minimized them. He really speaks so well of the people he loves. In some ways, I almost feel like I know them, but have only met some of them briefly.

We've talked about politics as well. It helps that we are on the same side of the fence. To this day, he's interested in politics and keeps up on things. He does an enormous amount of reading. I don't know how often he gets the *New York Times,* but he reads it pretty regularly and is always sharing articles and cutting things out.

Events and Stories

An interesting thing happened when Dr. Kennell turned 80. The people I worked with, our research coordinator, and her assistant, and myself managed to plan and carry out a surprise birthday party for Dr. Kennell. Mrs. Kennell was in on it, thank goodness. For a gift, we put together an album of written comments from various people. We contacted as many people as we could by going through his rolodex and asking if they would write something in honor of his 80th birthday. That was a really fun activity. Dr. Kennell's a smart guy, so to pull it off, we had a mini party to celebrate his birthday with some cupcakes, the kind of thing we did for everybody's birthday in the office. A couple of days later, we had the big surprise. It was out in the atrium in the BRB. A lot of people came by to celebrate knowing John Kennell. I think they were equally excited to know Mrs. Peggy Kennell. It was for both of them as much as for Dr. Kennell.

Grant writing is very stressful. He and I have written a few grants together, and I have some very nice memories of writing those. As you can imagine when you are trying to put together 30 to 40 pages of grant material, you have to spend a lot of time at work, and you rely on one another, along with other people, to get everything together. No matter what we would do, it always seemed there was pressure at the last minute, always rushing around. In the old days, which weren't that long ago, everything had to get mailed in; no computer submissions. You had to print it all and make multiple copies.

One of my fondest memories of writing a grant with Dr. Kennell happened when my daughter was 3. It was due in the late winter, a time when my husband, a CPA, is very busy, and I become like a single parent. My boys were older, 16 and 13. I could leave them alone while I was doing all this extra work, but I didn't want to leave my 3-year-old with her brothers for extended periods. She often came to the office with me, and I remember being there after dark with her, and working quite late into the evening. Dr. Kennell would be there along with our research coordinator at the time, Kirsten Brooks, who had tons of energy and was a wonderful person. We would be trying to get things pulled together and papers would be traveling back and forth between Kirsten xeroxing, and me typing things on the computer and correcting mistakes. Dr. Kennell would be in his office with my little girl on his lap, reading her stories. She was so happy to come to work with mom because she had the undivided attention of this wonderful caring individual, who would listen to her stories and who'd watch her draw pictures. This fond memory showed a side of Dr. Kennell that made him a wonderful person to work with.

There were many trials and tribulations of research. One time, we were told that a lot of people would be moving into our area so we'd been trying to clean up and have empty offices and empty cubicles for the new people. We'd been working for weeks and months to get people to come and take empty filing cabinets and to move old computer equipment that had been left by unknown individuals. Finally, I found the phone number of somebody who would come to pick up this stuff. I was eagerly waiting for it to happen. Then I came to work one day and the whole place looked different. The filing cabinets were gone, all the old computers were gone, everything was gone, including the computer that had all our data on it from our most recent project. I called Dr. Kennell at home and asked whether he knew anything about it. He said somebody came in with a bunch of big strong movers and dollies and moving equipment and started taking things out. He was told they were taking things because someone else needed the space. I said they took our computer with all our data on it. I wasn't too concerned because I knew we had everything on back up on zip disks. Then I looked and those were gone as well! So I was frantic until I got hold of the woman in charge and managed to track down the computer in the service center of Case Western Reserve. In a building off campus, in an area that had stacks and stacks of old abandoned computer equipment, I was able to find our computer with our data still on it.

Dr Kennell really believes in physical exercise. He quietly goes about it. I think he has been running for as long as I've known him. I don't know when he started jogging, although, I'm not sure he jogs on the road anymore. He would run through his neighborhood wherever that happened to be. So if he was at a conference in Germany, he'd be out running. If he was in a conference in Portugal, he'd find a place to get out of the hotel and go running. He used to run in Houston when he went once a month to meet about our study. Sometimes in Cleveland Heights, he ran in the streets if the snow wasn't clear on the sidewalks, or if it was after dark and the street lights would illuminate the streets. One time, Mrs. Kennell was out of town. Dr. Kennell went out jogging and he tripped and fell. I know because he came to work the next day and could hardly move his hands because his wrists were so swollen. They certainly didn't look good from what I could see. I don't know how he managed to get himself shaved and dressed that day the way his wrists were. When Mrs. Kennell came home, she had the same reaction and took him to the emergency room. I think one wrist was badly sprained, the other was broken. He had a cast on the broken wrist for a while, and had to do quite a bit of physical therapy to get the range of motion back in his wrist.

Early Events and Stories

When Dr. Kennell was a young pediatrician here at Rainbow, he was in charge of high-risk deliveries. There was no such thing as neonatology then, no neonatologists. If there was a delivery that appeared to be high risk for the baby in any way, they would call in the pediatrician on call. Dr. Kennell has memories of coming from Rainbow into those deliveries and having a baby handed to him that was in distress and not doing very well. So you're in the delivery room, and the mother has just had a Caesarean. Where do you go to revive a newborn? He talks about taking the newborn into a broom closet. There was no place near the delivery room on the 7th floor of MacDonald House. So he would take the newborn and go into this broom closet, surrounded by cleaning supplies. There, he'd work on the baby because he didn't think he could make it all the way to Rainbow and have the baby survive. I remember him showing me that awful broom closet. It's not there anymore.

This story demonstrates the self-control and calm demeanor that, to me, is Dr. Kennell. I've never seen him lose his temper or raise his voice, and this is an example of a time when he came as close as any. His family was on vacation in the U.S., and went to the beach for the day. He remembers that his children were fairly young and they had brought friends along. He stressed to everyone, "Do not close the trunk of the car because the car keys are in my pants pocket and I'm putting my clothes in the trunk of the car while we all go swimming." They went swimming, had a wonderful time and were exhausted. When they returned to the car, the trunk was closed. This was in the days before cell phones. What Dr. Kennell told me is that his kids say he said, "Oh Golly" about a million times. That was Dr. Kennell losing his temper.

Matthew

Dr. Kennell has taken family vacations, even with the kids as adults, so some of the grandchildren have been included. I think they went to Portugal not that many years ago. My area of expertise is families and the development of families. I think it's interesting to hear about Dr. Kennell's grandson, Matthew. He has graduated from college and is looking ahead to graduate school, careers, and many things that are similar to the interests and activities of his grandfather.

I think that's very nice. Matthew is very political, very involved in the Democratic Party at his university, and interested in international issues and events. While going through school, he was very athletic and very involved with his soccer teams, so things that are near and dear to Dr. Kennell have gone through the generations to his grandson, and that's a very nice thing. I hear that Matthew is a very well-liked individual, meets all different kinds of people, and connects with people of all different ages and cultural backgrounds. That reminds me of his grandpa, and that's interesting as well. I never met him, but I feel like I know him. His two younger grandchildren aren't grown up yet. I hear about them and their athletic abilities, and what a great dad and mom they have. He speaks with great pride about his family, and with humility too. But that's what he's like.

Note: Quotations were taken from unpublished interviews conducted by Mary Hellerstein, MD on September 27, 2007 and March 12, 2008.)

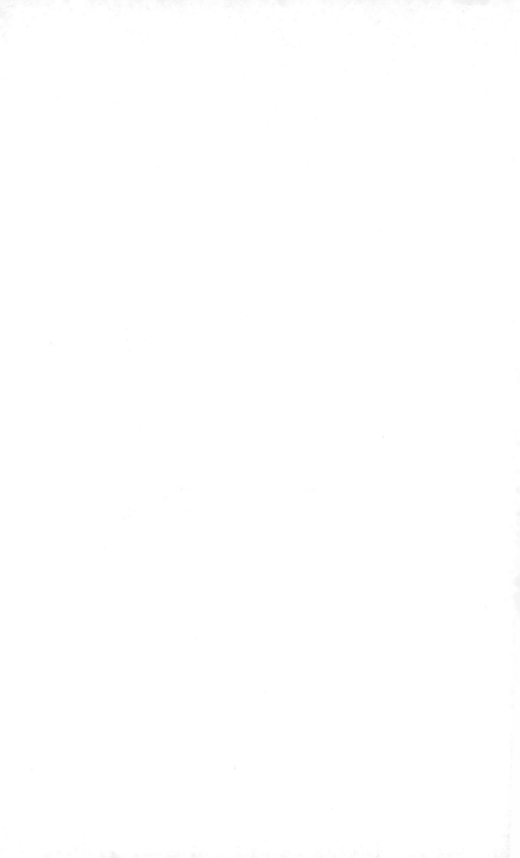

THE KENNELL FAMILY

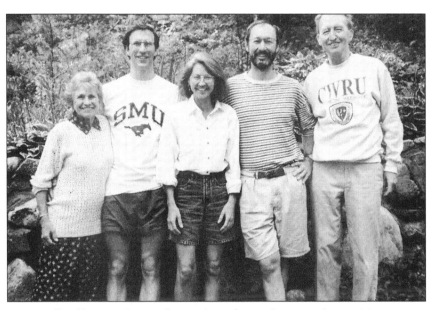

THE KENNELL FAMILY; PEGGY, JACK, SUSAN, DAVE AND JOHN; 1995

PEGGY KENNELL

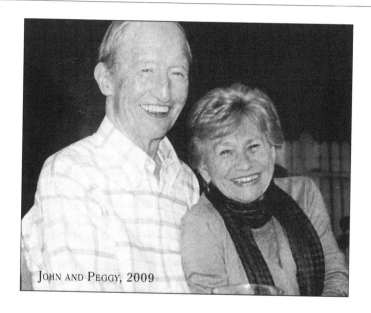

JOHN AND PEGGY, 2009

John and Margaret (Peggy) Kennell were married for 63 years. They had three children and five grandchildren. In December 2011, Peggy Kennell, and the three children of John and Peggy, recorded a conversation about John and what he means to them. The following information is taken from that recording.

Peggy was a pediatric nurse when she met John in 1946, working with a team led by Dr. Robert E. Gross, who was a pioneer in cardiovascular surgery on children at Boston Children's Hospital. She describes their meeting as follows; "The nursing school was having a dance and we were asked to invite young men. I was wheeling a patient through a ward when I noticed a new young doctor, a handsome man. I stopped to talk with him for a few minutes and asked if he would like to come to the dance. He said he would." That was the beginning of their romance.

Peggy knew from the beginning that John was the one. She said he was a very interesting person. He was attracted to history, politics, nature, and the world around him. She described him as gentle and kind. They had to be frugal, so, for entertainment, they took hikes together and went to the beach. In 1947, John left for Navy duty, but they met on weekends in New York and Washington D.C.

John and Peggy were married in 1949, while he was still in the Navy. They lived in Norfolk for a few months, and then returned to Boston, where John was the chief resident in pediatrics. Peggy continued to work as a surgical nurse until one month before their first child, David, was born. In 1952, a group of Harvard pediatricians were recruited to Cleveland, including Fred Robbins and William Wallace. Drs. Robbins and Wallace were asked to bring faculty with them and they invited John Kennell to join the group of seven or eight faculty members who moved to Cleveland and joined Western Reserve University. Peggy said they considered this a wonderful opportunity for John. He soon became chief of the Babies and Children's Hospital premature nursery and a specialist in neonatology.

Peggy thought John was happiest when he was teaching medical students and caring for mothers while being director of the family clinic at Babies and Children's Hospital. Spending a sabbatical year in London (July 1966 to July 1967) was a highlight for the Kennell family. John worked at the Great Ormond Street Hospital for Sick Children. This sabbatical year was the beginning of their desire to do more traveling and see the world. Upon John's return to Cleveland, he and his close colleague, Dr. Marshal Klaus, began their research studies on bonding and attachment.

Peggy said that John was very busy with his work, but always interested in his family and very proud of his children. As parents, they had the same values and similar expectations for their children. John loved reading bedtime stories and cherished vacations with his family. They especially enjoyed camping trips and going to Cape Cod. When the children were grown John and Peggy often traveled abroad where John was invited to lecture. They were able to develop many long-lasting friendships through their extensive travels and these trips greatly enhanced their lives.

DAVID, SUSAN, AND JACK

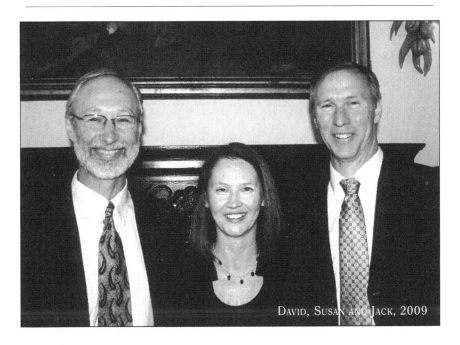

DAVID, SUSAN AND JACK, 2009

David

David Kennell was born in 1952, when John was almost 30 years old, the same age his father had been when he was born. David said he was impressed with his father's conversations about the children's hospital and the problems of poor people. He believes this is what led him into the field of public policy and health care, a field in which he has now become a leader.

David, like his father and grandparents, did his undergraduate work at the University of Rochester. He majored in public policy, a new field at the time. He then went to UC Berkeley graduate school, where he trained in public policy analysis, a program set up by the Ford Foundation that recognized the need for more experts in this field.

David currently heads a firm with 20 employees; its main focus is on Medicare and military health care plans. He works with many younger people, and he likens this to his father's work with medical students.

David remembers that his father talked about how talented many students were, how important it is to teach, and to recognize that some will achieve great things and others will not, and that it is always important to provide positive encouragement. David has found this to be his own experience as a mentor within his company.

Susan

Susan, the middle child and only daughter, was born at MacDonald House in Cleveland in 1953. MacDonald House is a maternity hospital where John did much of his research. Susan says that what stood out for her was John's continuing interest in the vulnerable, and this has impacted her career. She graduated from Ohio University with a degree in special education and a minor in anthropology. She also obtained a Master's degree from the University of Chicago. She wanted to work with families with abused children, and currently practices as a psychiatric counselor in Evanston, Illinois. She wanted to empower people, something that her father was very good at doing.

Susan knew that her father could appreciate both "simple" and "grand" things in people. He was as interested in the "simple things" as he was in the "grand things."

She described him as a "graceful" man with an ability to listen to people and make them feel important.

Susan went to Guatemala with John on one of his research trips there. She said that she was interested in the cultural issues, less so in the science.

She has continued her focus on clinical work to help people stay attached, and especially to help those with chronic illness and grief issues. This latter emphasis may be attributed to her observations of her father sitting with parents who had lost a baby. He did this every Monday night for many years, just sitting and listening. Susan says she modeled her work on her father's unique ability to listen carefully.

Susan described her close relationship with her own son, now 28 years old, and her two stepsons, ages 30 and 32. She says that John had a profound impact on his adult grandsons. He listened to them, rather than talking about himself. He often took out his pen and note cards and took notes related to what they said. This made people feel important.

Susan further described her father as "a man of little temper, gentle, and with a good sense of humor." She continues, "Everyone loved his sense of humor." He also was an early feminist. She recalled attending a meeting in which all the participants were female, except John, who sat and listened while the women led the meeting. She saw him as very different from men in "today's paternalistic society." She said, "He understood about suffering and power. He did not have to be the archetypal male."

Jack

John Carlyle Kennell was born in 1960. At age five, he announced that he would be known as Jack Kennell. Jack noted that his father was very busy, yet made time to take the family on camping vacations, and that is when Jack developed a love for the outdoors and for biology. His father was always very supportive of his interests. When John took him to meet his own mentor, Charles Janeway, Dr. Janeway gave Jack a book on biology.

When Jack was in high school, John arranged for him to meet Jay Rosenblatt, who did laboratory work, studying animal bonding in rats. Jack remembered that there were many faculty living in their neighborhood, and John encouraged his children to meet and talk with them. These interactions were influential in Jack's decision to become a research scientist.

Jack followed in the family footsteps to the University of Rochester, where he studied plants. Later, he went to Iowa State for his Master's degree, and obtained a PhD from the University of Florida in plant pathology. His research interests are in molecular biology, and is now a Full Professor at Saint Louis University. Like his father, he enjoys interacting with students. Jack explained that John made students feel important and had a teaching style of telling long stories to make a point. Jack said he is aware that he does the same thing. He also said that John would brag about the "smallest thing we did." They sometimes didn't want to tell their father about accomplishments because they were embarrassed by his telling his friends about them.

Jack appreciated the way John thrived on keeping up with contemporary events. He rarely missed the *Today Show,* or the *MacNeil/Lehrer News Hour* (now the *News Hour*), and subscribed to two daily newspapers. He was also a regular watcher of *Saturday Night Live,* and liked to have knowledge of the skits that were being performed. An avid believer in exercise, John rarely missed his nightly jog around the block.

All three of the children mentioned their father's strong work habits. Dave said, "I think we've all picked upon his work ethic" and learned from him that "to succeed, you have to apply yourself." Dave also remarked that "the collegiality in his career was impressive. He was happy to work with people with complementary skills." The message was that "you get more done by working with others." The Kennell family seems to exemplify these traits. Peggy and John beautifully complemented one another through the many years they spent together. It was evident by listening to the recording made by his family that his children care deeply for each other and their parents.

EULOGIES

JACK HORWITZ, MD

We were always aware that, above all, John loved, treasured, and was so proud of Peggy and their children.

How can you describe, in a few words, all the components that made John's achievements so special; gentleman, gentle man, doctor, educator, scholar, researcher, and advocate? There is a Yiddish phrase that is used to describe a very special person; "He is a real *mensh*." This definition, from Les Rosten's book, *The Joys of Yiddish*, really fits:

> A *mensh* is someone of consequence; -someone to admire
> and emulate, someone of noble character. "Now, there is a
> *real* mensh!"

John was, in every way, a real *mensh*.

I had the great privilege of knowing John for 51 years. I met him in 1962, when I started my residency in pediatrics at Babies and Children's Hospital in Cleveland.

A remarkable colleague! Although, he had many challenges and frustrations, in all those 51 years, I never once heard him say anything more vulgar than "gosh" or "darn"!

I will concentrate mainly on the earlier part of John's history-making career, and the lasting contributions he made to the education and attitude of thousands of medical students, pediatric residents, and nurses.

Most of you already know John was a very proud graduate of the University of Rochester School of Medicine. When he completed his residency in pediatrics at Boston Children's Hospital in 1952, he was recruited as a general pediatrician to Western Reserve University and Babies and Children's Hospital by the new chairman of pediatrics, Dr. William Wallace, who knew John from Boston. The medical school wanted Bill Wallace to build a strong research orientation for the department, and so recruiting talented sub-specialists became the focus. But John, a general pediatrician, was amongst the first chosen by Wallace. Several of these early sub-specialists went on to distinguished careers and leadership in American pediatrics. But of Wallace's initial recruits, John is probably *the* most well-known, worldwide.

John was immediately given a few "simple" responsibilities; the first full-time director of the first and newly-built "Premie Unit" at Babies and Children's. That was quite a task for this newly appointed assistant professor, fresh out of his residency training! John helped make this unit thrive and lead it to be the neonatal service that attracted new partners and then successors, Marshall Klaus, Avroy Fanaroff, Richard Martin, and Michelle Walsh; a unit that is now world-renowned and respected as amongst the very best of the best.

John was also appointed Director of the Pediatric Outpatient Clinic. That meant he was also the director of the Pediatric Emergency at University Hospital, in the basement of Lakeside Hospital. Also, as Director of the Pediatric Emergency, he became the Director of the Poison Control Center for NE Ohio. This was located in the residents' office / bedroom / library of the Pediatric Emergency Ward.

To make sure he was not bored, John was also named Director of the Family Clinic. Soon, he took on a little more responsibility as Director of the Newborn Nurseries at MacDonald Women's Hospital. Oh, I nearly forgot, he was also the Pediatric Residency Training Program Director at Babies and Children's.

Of course, Rainbow Hospital, at that time located in South Euclid, wanted a Pediatrician in charge, so you need not doubt who filled that role. As a general pediatric consultant, John had a small private referral practice as well.

Let's review what John brought to the plate in just a few of those administrative, patient care, and educational responsibilities;

John's words on the Premie Unit:

> I had not expected to be doing things with prematures when I came to Cleveland, but I think I was helped by two forces. One was this glass wall that let you see into the nursery, whereas most nurseries had been hidden, or perhaps had just one little peephole. And then there was a very nice and cooperative head nurse, Jane Cable, and she and I were talking about changing things. All the writings about premature care advised that absolutely no parent should ever be permitted in the nursery. So, Jane and I arranged for the parents to come into the nursery, and it was usually the mothers, and at first we just had them come by and stand by the isolette, and then it progressed to where they could hold the baby and then feed the baby.

Here John showed that, despite his quiet, dignified exterior, he could be tough and prevail to bring about what amounted to revolutionary change for something he believed in. Something that would be of great benefit to children and their families and which, through research, he strived to prove.

Within a few years John, with the enthusiastic support of Babies and Children's Nursing Director, Miss Dalia Zemaityte, did the unthinkable—they persuaded the hospital to permit parents to stay with their children in the hospital. Later, all visiting hours were abolished. Nationally, they were severely challenged, even ridiculed, but in their enthusiastic but humble way, John and Dalia were spectacularly successful and changed the world for hospitalized infants and children and their families.

John taught us to understand the disease that was affecting a child, and to treat that carefully and specifically where possible. But he also taught us not to neglect the big picture; the family, culture, and environment. He held that every child deserved the best possible treatment, irrespective of financial or social status, race, religion or tradition, but to be aware and deal with the roles these factors all play in managing a child and family's health and well-being.

PAMELA DAVIS, PhD, MD

John Kennell was an extraordinary professor. He taught by his textbook, he taught on rounds, he taught in the hallways, and he probably introduced more medical students to research than any other single individual at our School of Medicine—and that's saying something. He was a clinical investigator ahead of the time when it became fashionable. More important, perhaps, is that he taught us the value of the human element in medicine; how a gentler entry into the world made children more confident and aware, and how that gentler entry could be achieved by simple human contact. He was an icon.

He embodied the kinder, gentler, human element. My geriatric colleagues tell me that as we age, we become more like ourselves. As John aged, he was a beacon of joy, smiling at everyone and greeting his friends, gracious and well-mannered, self-effacing, and loving toward his family. In my mind's eye, I will see him on the dance floor at the Silver Grille, with his wife. He is smiling and just swaying a bit to the music, but he is out on the floor to make her happy. He loved her very much.

May it be given to all of us to be happy, to love and be loved, and to change a part of the world for the good. John did.

Dean, Case Western Reserve School of Medicine

KAREN OLNESS, MD

D ear Peggy, Susan, David, Jack, Kennell grandchildren, other family and friends,

I first met John Kennell in the 70s when he came to speak in Minneapolis. Like many of my pediatric generation, I was in awe of him. After I had the opportunity to meet with him, I was amazed and also happy to know that he was so kind, so humble, so caring, and so generous with his time. He listened to young colleagues and encouraged them. He thought carefully about our questions and he was an outstanding role model for generations of developmental behavioral pediatricians, and for health care providers in all specialties.

John and I became close friends. We joked about the fact that we were the only members of our division to carry our lunches to Rainbow. John had a green lunch bag, mine was blue. Invariably, his contained two sandwiches and fruit, and mine had one sandwich and fruit. Several years ago, Mary Hellerstein and I began working on a biography of John. John patiently gave us more than 30 recorded interviews, which were transcribed as a labor of love by one of our fellows, Shanna Kralovic. The biography was nearly done two years ago. One day in October 2011, I sat with John in his office, going through the detailed scrapbooks of his early life, and selecting photos to be included in the biography. These included his meticulous baby book, assembled by his loving mother. John laughed as he reminisced and shared more stories. And at his 90th birthday party, in January 2012, I was able to give him a draft copy of the biography. That evening, I remember he and Peggy danced to the piano music of Howard Hall.

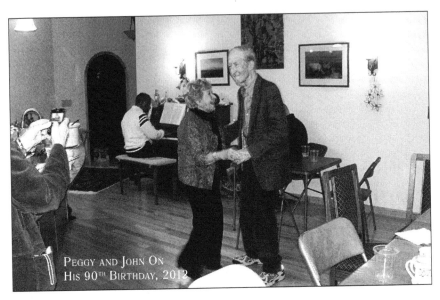

PEGGY AND JOHN ON HIS 90TH BIRTHDAY, 2012

John's accomplishments and contributions to benefit mothers and children were enormous and in multiple areas. He deserves gratitude from families in the U.S. and around the world for his leadership in emphasizing the importance of early mother-infant attachment, in promoting generous parental visitation for hospitalized children, for documenting the grief that parents of newborns suffer and pioneering bereavement groups for them, for facilitating child-life programs in hospitals, and for documenting the value of doulas in supporting mothers through labor and delivery.

He was a devoted and outstanding educator, participating in medical student groups until just a few years ago. He was also a leader in global child health education, urging the American Academy of Pediatrics to develop global child health programs in the 80s. He served on the first task force to begin that process. He taught in the "Preparation for International Health Service" seminar series for our medical students and residents for 18 years, and he also taught in the annual five-day workshop on "Management of disasters: Focus on children and families" for 12 years. In this workshop, he taught about how children perceive death at differing developmental stages, and ways to help bereaved children.

He was a member of the standing committee of the International Pediatric Association during the 90s, and he was a Board Member of Health Frontiers for 22 years. One of those board meetings took place in Hawaii, where we visited a new hospital on the Big Island. The hospital had a state-of-the-art birthing unit. I remember the excitement of the nursing staff there when they realized that John Kennell was visiting them.

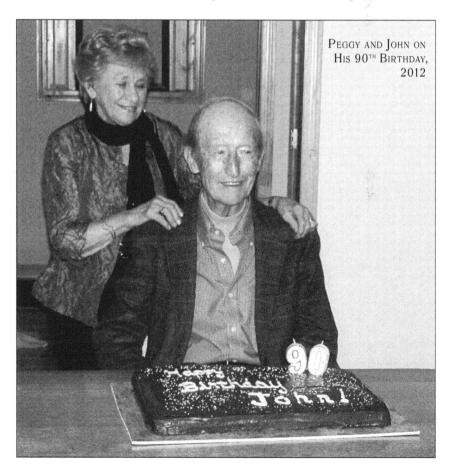

PEGGY AND JOHN ON HIS 90TH BIRTHDAY, 2012

Many of his educational efforts reflected his generous volunteer service. He was President of the Society of Developmental Behavioral Pediatrics in 1991, and he subsequently chaired a committee to work with the American Board of Pediatrics in formalizing the subspecialty of developmental behavioral pediatrics. He received many awards, including the Aldrich Award given by the American Academy of Pediatrics

John Kennell was a thoughtful and gracious person, never failing to send congratulatory notes to students, colleagues, and families about achievements. These were carefully handwritten and regarded as treasures by the recipients. John was usually positive and hopeful, even in difficult situations. Very rarely, he would use his strongest expletive, "son of a gun."

John's teaching impacted many foreign trainees at Rainbow. I am closing with some statements sent to me by former fellows from other countries. They convey the essence of this wonderful man better than anything I could say.

From Dr. Pulsuk Siripul (Professor, School of Nursing, Khon Kaen University)

"Thank you for telling me about Dr. Kennell's passing. He is a great person with his kindness and gentleness still staying in my memory. I knew his work and I feel so honored to have met him and I had a good time in learning from him. Please pass my high respect and warm friendship from Thailand. May God lead his spirit to heaven."

From Dr. Saleh Al Salehi (Director General Hospital Programs, Saudi Arabia)

"I am very sorry this loss. My deepest condolences for his family and friends. Please send my condolences to his wife. Unfortunately, I can't attend."

"He was the most passionate pediatrician I ever met. He was giving without limits, and never said, 'sorry, I can't help,' especially to foreign trainees like myself.

God bless his soul."

Regards,

Saleh

From Dr. Niramol Pajanasoontorn (Professor, Psychiatry Department, Khon Kaen University)

Please tell Peggy that I am so sorry. John was so kind to me and I want to say thanks to him and my deepest sympathy and sadness with his family.

Niramol

Dear John,

What your students and patients remember and admire and emulate is that you took time to listen to them, that you nurtured them, and that you cared. Most did not know the extent of your fame, and you didn't tell them. You remained true to yourself, embodying humility, generosity and, above all, love.

Thank you!

REFERENCES

Ainsfield, E., Casper, V., Nozyce, M., & Cunningham, N. (1990). Does infant carrying promote attachment? *Child Development, 61,* 1617-1627.

Ainsfield, E., Curry, M.A., Hales, D.J., Kennell, J.H., Klaus, M.H., Lipper, E., O'Connor, S., Siegel, E., & Sosa, R. (1983). Maternal-infant bonding: A joint rebuttal. *Pediatrics, 72,* 569-572.

Barnett, C.R., Leiderman, P.H., Grobstein, R., & Klaus, M.H. (1970). Neonatal separation: The maternal side of interactional deprivation. *Pediatrics, 45,* 197.

Brazelton, T.B. (1961). Psychophysiological reactions of the neonate. II. Effects of maternal medication on the neonate and his behavior. *Pediatrics, 58,* 513.

Hales, D.J., Lozoff, B., Sosa, R., & Kennell, J.H. (1977). Defining the limits of the maternal sensitive period. *Developmental Medicine & Child Neurology, 19,* 454-461.

Horwitz, S.J., Doershuk, C.F., & Edey, N.C. (2007). *For the children.* Cleveland: University Hospital Health Systems, Inc.

INFDC (1995). *The Santa Maria Cauque study: Health and survival of Mayan Indians under deprivation, Guatemala by Leonardo Mata in Community-Based Longitudinal Nutrition and Health Studies: Classical Examples from Guatemala, Haiti and Mexico.*

Kennell, J.H. (1980). Are we in the midst of a revolution? *American Journal of Diseases of Childhood, 134,* 303-310.

Kennell, J.H. (2003). Benefits of a doula present at the birth of a child. *Journal of Developmental & Behavioral Pediatrics, 24,* 195-198.

Kennell, J.H., & Chickering, D.C. (1961). Experience with a medical school family study. *Journal of Medical Education, 36,* 1649-1716.

Kennell, J.H., Jerauld, R., Wolf, H., Chesler, D., Kreger, N., McAlpine, W., Steffa, M., & Klaus, M. (1974). Maternal behavior one year after early and extended post-partum contact. *Developmental Medicine and Child Neurology, 16,* 172-179.

Kennell, J.H., & Klaus, M.H. (1979). Early mother-infant contact. *Bulletin Menninger Clinic, 43,* 69-78.

Kennell, J., Klaus, M., McGrath, S., Robertson, S., & Hinkley C. (1991). Continuous Emotional Support During Labor in a US Hospital. *Journal of American Medical Association, 265,* 2197-2201.

Kennell, J.H., Slyter, H., & Klaus, M.H. (1970). Mourning response of parents to the death of a newborn. *New England Journal of Medicine, 283,* 344-349.

Klaus, M. (2000). *Personal interview by LM Gartner for the Oral history project of the American Academy of Pediatrics.* p 57. Retrieved from: www2.aap.org/sections/perinatal/pdf/Klausoralhistory.pdf

Klaus, M.H., Clements, J.A., & Havel, R.J. (1961). Composition of surface-active material isolated from beef lung. *Proceedings of the National Academy of Sciences, 47*(11), 1858-1859.

Klaus, M.H., Jerauld, R., Kreger, M.C., McAlpine, W., Steffa, M., & Kennell, J.H. (1972). Maternal attachment: Importance of the first post-partum days. *New England Journal of Medicine, 286,* 460-463.

Klaus, M.H., & Kennell, J.H. (1976). *Maternal-infant bonding: The impact of early separation or loss on family development.* St. Louis: Mosby.

Klaus, M.H., & Kennell, J.H. (1982). *Parent-infant bonding: The impact of early loss or separation on family development.* St. Louis: Mosby.

Klaus, M.H., & Kennell, J.H. (1983). *Bonding: The beginnings of parent-infant attachment.* St. Louis, MO: Mosby.

Klaus, M. H., & Kennell, J.H. (2004). Parents in the preterm nursery and subsequent evolution of care. *Neo Reviews, 5,* 397-405.

Klaus, M.H., Kennell, J.H., & Klaus, P.H. (2002, 2012). *The doula book.* Cambridge, MA: Perseus.

Klaus, M.H., Kennell, J.H., Plumb, N., & Zuehlke, S. (1970). Human maternal behavior at first contact with her young. *Pediatrics, 46,*187-192.

Klaus, M.H., Kennell, J.H., Robertson, S.S., & Sosa, R. (1986). Effects of social support during parturition on maternal and infant morbidity. *British Medical Journal, 293,* 585-587.

Klaus, M.H., Trause, M.A., & Kennell, J.H. (1975). Does human maternal behavior after delivery show a characteristic pattern. *CIBA Foundation Symposium, 33,* 69-85.

Landry, S.H., McGrath, S., Kennell, J.H., Martin, S., & Steelman L. (1998). The effect of doula support during labor on mother-infant interactions at 2 months. *Pediatric Research, 43,* 13A.

McGrath, S.K., & Kennell, J.H. (2008). A randomized controlled trial of continuous labor support for middle-class couples: Effect on cesarean delivery rates. *Birth, 35,* 92-97.

McGrath, S.K., Kennell, J.H., Suresh, M., Moise, K., & Hinckley, C. (1999). Doula support vs. epidural analgesia: Impact on cesarean rates. *Pediatric Research, 45,* 16A.

Murdock, G.P., & White, G.R. (1969). Standard cross-cultural sample. *Ethology, 8,* 329-369.

Raphael, D. (1973). *The tender gift: Breastfeeding.* Englewood Cliffs, NJ: Prentice-Hall.

Ringler, N.M., Kennell, J.H., Jarvella, R., Navojosky, B.J., & Klaus, M.H. (1975). Mother-to-child speech at two years–Effects of increased early postnatal contact. *Journal of Pediatrics, 86*(1), 141-144

Ringler, N., Trause, M.A., Klaus, M.H., & Kennell, J.H. (1978). The effects of extra postpartum contact and maternal speech patterns on children's IQ's, speech and language comprehension at five. *Child Development, 49,* 862-865.

Sosa, R., Kennell, J.H., Klaus, M., & Urrutia, J.J. (1976). The effect of early mother-infant contact on breast feeding, infection and growth. *CIBA Foundation Symposium, 45,* 179-193.

Sosa, R., Kennell, J., Klaus, M., Robertson, S., & Urrutia, J. (1980). The effect of a supportive companion on perinatal problems, length of labor, and mother-infant interaction. *New England Journal of Medicine, 303,* 597-600.

Urrutia, J.J., Sosa, R., Kennell, J.H., & Klaus, M. (1979). Prevalence of maternal and neonatal infections in a developing country: Possible low-cost preventive measures. *CIBA Foundation Symposium, 77,* 171-186.

APPENDICES

Eng 3b   John Kennell
December 12, 1938   II L Period

SELLING MAGAZINES

Somehow or other, I was selling magazines. Somehow or other, I always was attracted by big, brightly colored advertisements proclaiming, "You, too, can make Christmas money, buy several bicycles, etc." Somehow or other, I had been encouraged to accept the offer, possibly through my parents urging, possibly through the dreadful realization that it was December, Christmas was coming, and I was financially at a loss. Somehow or other, I had finally arrived at the dangerous period in magazine selling where relatives had run out and one has to resort to the magnificent technique of salesmanship.

Every free hour I spent plodding the streets, first choosing only the more inviting houses but now down to a door-to-door canvas. Rain and shine, washday and holiday, winter and summer I worked. I adopted the absolutely flawless sales technique, in a book, of a hundred or more successful salesmen and prominent business men who had gotten their start with my magazine company. I memorized the speeches they used to positively clinch the sale. Maybe Buffalonians were different, maybe my appearance was repulsive. Something was the matter.

The book said nothing about what to do when people came to the door, sleepily, in bathrobes, haughtily, with the news they already had the magazines or, angrily, with a vacuum cleaner in one hand, a dust rag in the other, and a curse on their lips. They came, threateningly, with serious intent to murder the next salesman, no matter what his commodity or sales talk. Or, as was the case, nine times out of ten—what to do when—even though you wore your thumb out ringing, the people inside carried on a lively conversation supplemented by, "Shush—there's another peddler"—and you dressed up just the way J.J. Johnson, a prominent New York insurance salesman, said he "absolutely wowed" his customers.

Then, too, dogs presented a menacing problem, especially in flats. I would enter the hallway of a flat and there encounter two bells and two doors. I tried all systems—even hoped the law of averages would assist me, but invariably I picked the wrong bell. I would ring the bell, straighten my tie, stand before the door I hoped would open, put on a cheery smile, arrange the magazines all over the front of me until I looked like a surrealistic painting of a wall paper exhibit, and prepared an appropriate speech. I would hear footsteps coming, the hand on the doorknob, and then the door—the other door—would swing open, knock me down and send my magazines flying. Then, always, to add insult to injury, a huge mastiff would stand on me, smack his lips and drool all over me and my fresh clean magazines (another surefire secret for success), and prepare to devour me. Then, unless I had a sympathetic customer, he would laugh, while the dog mauled me and chewed my clothes, and say the dog was playful, wouldn't hurt a flea or other disparaging remarks made especially unbearable because salesmen must laugh at their customer's jokes.

When I would see the dog preparing for the kill, I would attempt to ward off the blow only to be rewarded by a broken arm and an angry scowl from the customer. Finally, the dog would be convinced I was dead and go away. Then, if I was still able, I would present my badly tattered magazines and not make a sale. Never did I make a sale to one of that type of customer, even though I encountered that type by the thousands.

Then, among the steady customers, there were always the people who couldn't pay until next week because the money was upstairs, even though you had walked ten blocks to collect. However, there were some really grand people you finally found, people whose genial encouragement more than made up which helped the salesman along his way. Selling magazines, with all its discouragements, is a grand experience, and at the end of the salesman's road to success lies the happiness—the extreme happiness—which a salesman gains from the really true friendships he makes along the way.

VALEDICTORY

By John Kennell

Tonight, we say farewell to our school days in Bennett. Tomorrow, we set forth anew—some to continue academic work in institutions which provide further training for life's work, many set out more directly on their chosen vocations, all to apply the training that Bennett has given them, all to carry on in the Bennett spirit.

But tonight is ours together to look back over four years spent at Bennett—four years of learning the things which will be helpful–four years under the guidance of Mr. Farrar and his corps of capable and friendly assistants—four years of classes, of school plays, debates, sports, dances, assemblies—four years that we shall never forget—four years that have left an imprint on our lives that can never be erased.

True, the battles of Life will deeply affect us—but the influences of these four years will never completely be removed. We have emerged from the irresponsibilities of childhood to the grim realities of more adult life. Our philosophy has been developed. Our traits of character and personality are fairly well established. We have formed friendships that will endure. We have undergone experiences that will always remain in our memory. We have gained a spirit that will enable us to meet the adversities of later life. You, the Bennett faculty, have filled us with hopes and aspirations and yet you have tempered your optimism with words of caution. You have painted bright pictures but have softened them with shadows, lest we be disillusioned. We go forth with the spirit of the adventurer, for we believe that there is still work to be done in the world. Tomorrow, we go forth to do this work.

If we go to college, we shall struggle to keep bright the banner of Bennett High School, already placed in front lines by Bennett graduates who have preceded us.

If we go more immediately to join the ranks of the workers, we shall try to keep with us still the spirit of seekers after knowledge. We shall not close our minds with the close of our last formal scholastic examination.

And so—we say "farewell," it is not "goodbye," but rather "until we meet again." We will come back to Bennett in memory many times. Many times, lessons learned during high school days will help us meet the demands and changes, which are bound to come. While oft times the way has seemed hard, still we want our teachers to know that we are thankful for their efforts to assist us. As students, we have admired their abilities—as boys and girls, we have appreciated their personal interest in our joys and sorrow. We have appreciated their loyal friendships.

As we leave Bennett High School, we take with us the spirit of our Alma Mater—the spirit that has made our four years so profitable, so enjoyable—the same optimism expressed in our motto, "THE BEST IS YET TO BE."

THE JOHN H. KENNELL CHAIR IN CHILD PSYCHIATRY

Acceptance Speech by Dr. Kennell

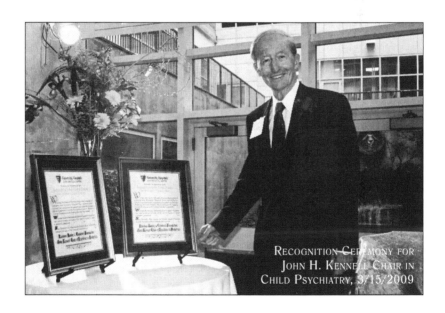

RECOGNITION CEREMONY FOR JOHN H. KENNELL CHAIR IN CHILD PSYCHIATRY, 3/15/2009

3/15/2009

It's a great honor to be here for this important event and to receive the endowed chair that has been generously given in my name. I want to express my gratitude to Pat Swenson and the public relations department, and everyone who directly or indirectly contributed to this honor tonight.

I have been exceptionally fortunate to have spent the last 57 years in such a supportive environment as that of Rainbow Babies and Children's Hospital. I'm also very grateful for the encouragement of my work and interests by the Rainbow Board, my research colleagues, the doctors, nurses, medical students, and support staff. This, of course, includes the love and support from all of my good friends—many of you are here tonight. And I especially thank my wife, Peggy, and our children, David, Susan, and Jack. I thank you all.

When I first came to Cleveland as a pediatrician in 1952, we were providing state-of-the-art care for premature babies, born at MacDonald Hospital, and cared for at what was called Babies and Children's, or B&C.

At that time, all of the preemies were lined up in isolates with bright lights, and touched only by nurses and physicians, wearing rubber gloves to avoid infections.

During that period, some obstetrics hospitals were not as familiar with care by a pediatrician after a baby was born. I remember many experiences with babies who were having trouble breathing, and I would often be called on the 8th floor of B&C, and would run all the way down the stairs to the maternity hospital, and then run up 7 floors to a large surgical amphitheatre. The nurses were clear from their orders that I could not enter the large room to help the sick baby and would direct me to a very small room. I would find mops hanging upside down with buckets on the floor in that tiny room. So, while focusing on resuscitating the babies, we would often find ourselves trying to ignore our feet getting into the buckets and the mops sometimes falling down. Thankfully, a well-outfitted facility was opened a year or two later.

During my career, I have continued to have a heightened interest in how to get and keep mothers and fathers together with their babies, to touch them, and have contact as early as possible.

In the 1950s, Head Nurse Jane Cable, in the premature nursery, teamed up with me in carefully allowing and supporting mothers into the nursery to be with their neonates. At first, after they carefully scrubbed, the mothers might sit next to the baby and look at the baby... then they might touch the baby's foot or stroke the baby... and days or weeks later, might feed the baby, sometimes on their lap, usually with a nurse present. The mother's seemed *so* appreciative, and we noticed that not only did the parents seem less anxious and scared about their tiny and sick baby, but that the babies themselves thrived and appeared to develop better.

In 1967, Marshall Klaus and I joined up to carry our research together as we shared the same interests in the importance of contact between mothers and fathers with their infants within the first hour of life. I feel that I share this honor tonight with Marshall; and Marshall, would you please stand up so that you can be acknowledged.

Later on his wife, Phyllis, joined us with our publications, and would you please stand up as well?

At MacDonald House, Marshal and I began the first studies of early contact, or what we now call "bonding" of full-termed, healthy babies. The first contact between mother and baby at that time averaged much more than an hour after birth, compared to the present time, when early contact with the mother and inclusion of the father begins immediately after birth.

Another challenge was to allow parents to live in with their hospitalized child, and I well remember Scott Dowling's efforts in supporting me with this. The new Rainbow Babies and Children's Hospital willingly accommodated this change for all parents. My colleagues, Av Faneroff, Richard Martin, Maureen Hack, and others were also instrumental in encouraging this change. Once again, the Rainbow Board was forward thinking and supportive.

I would be remiss if I didn't also include my special colleagues; Karen Olness, who has given me endless encouragement and inspiration, and is a living example of how much can be accomplished for children in the world, and Susan McGrath, who has been so devoted with her planning, analysis, and publication skills, and she still works tirelessly with me. And Bobbie O'Bell, whose nursing and leadership skills were crucial for several research studies.

Terms like "kangaroo care" and the "doula" have become commonplace ideas and practices. We're pretty sure that there were times when some of our focus and efforts might have seemed like "crazy ideas," but nonetheless, the Board members and Hospital supported us. Eventually, we noticed that other hospitals around the country were emulating the practices of this hospital and its staff.

Members of the board, and their president, Kim Pesses, in essence, you were our doulas; our supportive partners in the development of these ideas and practices.

So now, the new neonatal unit will be an amazing innovation for other hospitals to emulate, and we are, again, going to be able to continue these efforts into the future for decades with the Chair endowment. Preemies today are surviving at weights we couldn't have fathomed. The physical contact is immediate. They are in a beautiful private room with soft lighting, so that the mothers and (sometimes fathers) may live in with their preemie for 3 or more months.

I look forward to learning of the advances that develop from this new facility. I am assured that Rainbow Babies and Children's Hospital will remain at the forefront of supporting secure attachment for families and babies.

Again, I want to thank all of you for coming tonight, for all of your loyalty, financial support, patience, and faith in these ideas that we hope promote the best care for babies and their families.

Most of all, I am forever grateful to the preemies, babies, children, and their parents that have taught us so much and helped us move their care forward. Because of this endowment, they can continue to keep teaching us and showing us about these important relationships for many years to come.

Thank you.

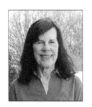

Karen Olness, MD, is Professor Emerita of Pediatrics, Global Health and Diseases at Case Western Reserve University and board certified in developmental behavioral pediatrics. She has worked in resource poor areas of the world over a 50 year period, with a focus on helping children in disasters. She worked with John Kennell for 24 years.

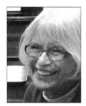

Carolyn Myers, PhD served in the Peace Corps in Thailand in the beautiful northern city of Chiang Mai. As a biochemist she subsequently joined the busy Division of Pediatric Pharmacology and Critical Care at Rainbow Babies and Children's Hospital in Cleveland, Ohio. Following retirement, Carolyn joined Karen Olness and Mary Hellerrstein in completing the preparation of this biography of Dr. John Kennell.

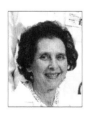

Mary Hellerstein, MD, graduated from Laurel School in 1939, and from Smith College in 1943. She graduated from the Western Reserve School of Medicine in 1949. Mary was a pediatrician in Cleveland for many years and worked at Rainbow Hospital and the Hough-Norwood Clinic for many years as well.

Made in the USA
San Bernardino, CA
22 February 2016